Voices of Alzheimer's

The Healing Companion: Stories for Courage, Comfort and Strength

Edited by

The Healing Project

www.thehealingproject.org

"Voices Of" Series Book No. 2

LaChancepublishing

LACHANCE PUBLISHING • NEW YORK

www.lachancepublishing.com

Publisher: LaChance Publishing LLC
            120 Bond Street
            Brooklyn, NY 11201
            www.lachancepublishing.com

All things have a beginning, although sometimes the journey from beginning to end is not always so clear and straightforward. While work on *Voices Of* began just two years ago, truth be told, the seeds were planted long ago by beloved sources. This book is dedicated to Jennie, Larry and Denise, who in the face of all things good and bad extended courage and support in excess. And especially to Richard, who taught us by the way he lived his life that anything is possible given enough time, hard work and love.

Contents

Part I: THE PARENTS

Part II: THE SPOUSES

Part III: THE GRANDPARENTS

Part IV: THE CAREGIVERS

Foreword

David Shenk

In these rich pages, you will find anger, acceptance, bewilderment, determination, compassion, and lots and lots of love. Alzheimer's is amongst the worst of afflictions, but it brings out the very best in people. Though I haven't yet had to face the disease in my own family, it has been my honor and privilege to be a part of the Alzheimer's community for almost a decade. There's plenty of loss and sadness, to be sure, but what really shines through is the well-spring of humanity. It is simply inspiring.

In my writing, filmmaking and speaking, I've made it my mission to help people better understand the disease. Families have an especially vexing experience if they don't know at least the fundamentals—what the disease does to the brain and how it travels around its various regions.

By the same token, though, no doctor or scientist or social worker or legal advisor can possibly have a clue about Alzheimer's until they've spent gobs of time with patients and their families. Office visits just don't convey the exploding reality of how this disease unravels actual lives. But these pages do. Here you will soak in not just the predictable heartache but also the eloquent landscape of decline. Each page evokes a common experience, and yet speaks to every person's unique mark on the earth.

Why read a book of such sad stories? Because the same book also provides a sharp lens into the world of lives well lived. And that is what we all seek, what we all strive for.

Brooklyn, New York
July, 2006

David Shenk is an award-winning, bestselling author and a contributor to *National Geographic*, *Harper's*, National Public Radio, *The New Yorker*, *Gourmet*, *Wired*, and *The American Scholar*. His most recent book, *The Forgetting*, won First Prize in the British Medical Association's Popular Medical Book Awards." Mr. Shenk speaks frequently on the history, biology and social urgency of Alzheimer's Disease and has advised the President's Council on Bioethics on dementia-related issues.

Introduction

I wanted to ask the people around me, "Would you please raise your hand if you feel as isolated as I do?" Walking the busy streets of Manhattan on a beautiful sunny day, I was surrounded by people but I'd never felt so alone. Just minutes before, my doctors had broken the news to me that I had a particularly aggressive form of breast cancer.

Since moving to New York from a small town in Rhode Island, I'd had my share of ups and downs but had always risen to the challenges that living and working in New York can bring. But on this summer afternoon, I felt as if the world was suddenly rushing past me while I seemed to be moving in slow motion along the crowded sidewalk, wondering how I was going to take the next step, the one I dreaded the most: how was I going to tell my twin sister Denise? How do you tell someone you love so much that you have cancer?

My sister and I are as close as only twins can be. Ever since I can remember, Denise has been my best friend, my greatest support, my closest confidante. She was always at my side as I built successful businesses in fashion, technology, and real estate. We had faced challenges together in the past, but cancer was new territory. As I reached for my cell phone, I shook my head at the thought that I'd have several similar calls to make. Telling my loved ones that I had cancer would be worse than hearing it myself.

But with a life of love and support behind us and uncertainty ahead, Denise and I did what we had always done: we got to work. There was much research to do and a short amount of time in which to do it: specialists to consult; doctors to interview; treatment plans to decide upon; hospitals to find. All complicated by time: all the while the clock was ticking, urging me to move forward.

I found that one of the first things I almost automatically began to look for, besides doctors, was a sense of connection. I needed to hear from other people who had gone through what I was experiencing, who truly understood what it meant and who might be able to help. I wasn't ready for a regular support group, and with surgery and treatment looming, I simply didn't have the time. But I am an avid reader, and I assumed that finding the personal stories of those who had gone through this ordeal before me would be relatively easy. There seemed to be a vacuum; almost nothing. Where were the *real people* to talk to? Where was the literature that wasn't just about the hardcore science of the disease?

There was one book that gave me great solace, *Just Get Me Through This* by Deborah Cohen and Robert A. Gelfand. It was more of a personal story, rather than a clinical one, and it created in me a desire for more stories that get to the heart of the emotional experience, that help the reader through it. In my limited time talking with other breast cancer patients, I knew there were countless others out there who needed to tell their stories—and to hear the stories of others as well. I decided that part of my own, ongoing healing process would be to find a way to bring people like me together, to create some kind of forum where these real stories could be shared.

First I had to find the doctors who would make the physical healing possible. From the beginning, I knew I wanted a female surgeon to handle my case, but as Denise and I did the research about the disease and its treatment, one doctor's name kept repeating:

Dr. Alexander Swistel, the Director of the Weill Cornell Breast Center at Weill Medical College at Cornell University. He wasn't in my insurance network, but after meeting with him I knew he would be the one. It was scary enough to go through this at all, let alone do it with a surgeon who didn't make me feel as comfortable as possible. Dr. Swistel put me at my ease, gave me confidence and made me feel that I was in good hands.

I also felt instant rapport with my oncologist Ellen Gold. Dr. Gold was frank and honest, while leaving me room to express my concerns. For many cancer patients, there's little time to bring up feelings between diagnosis and the start of treatment, much less have them addressed. The whole process moves so quickly, sometimes in a seeming trance, that the patient can feel as if she's being run through a healthcare assembly line with no chance to even firmly attach names to the faces of the many medical professionals responsible for her care. Dr. Gold always made me feel that there was time.

In addition to Denise, my family, my doctors, and my friends, what got me through that process were the little lies I told myself in order get my mind wrapped around the reality of my situation. I'd seen my pathology report, and I started to devour all the literature on the disease, selecting all of the information that would help me to put the best "spin" on my condition. There's so much information out there, so many statistics, reports and findings that I could always find something to latch onto that would allow me to continually push the scariest possibilities away.

But the initial pathology report was wrong. The corrected report I received soon after the first indicated the highest presence of Her-2 (human epidermal growth factor receptor), which results in significantly worse survival rates in patients because its presence can lead to an intense proliferation of cancer cells. Time stood still for me as I read this new report, and in that stillness I finally felt the full impact of my diagnosis. It was then that denial stopped working. It was then that I knew I'd need chemotherapy. Like so many women, the thought of losing my hair to chemotherapy brought it all crashing home, and as it is with many other patients, it was my turning point. Hitting that hard wall of reality, the time had come to finally face it and fight ... or not.

I chose to fight, and in making that choice my vision of community crystallized and *The Healing Project* was born. I'd already realized that having access to the real stories of real people would make the journey through breast cancer much easier to endure. My thoughts kept returning to that walk through Manhattan after I'd heard my diagnosis and that feeling I had of terrible loneliness. As sympathetic as friends and loved ones could be, I felt that no one could truly understand this journey except someone who had walked in the same shoes. As my surgery drew closer, I became convinced that getting and giving courage, comfort, and strength were as important as good medical care, and I became determined to help build a community for people like me who were undergoing the terribly isolating experience of dealing with a life-threatening disease. This would be *The Healing Project*'s mission: to become a bridge across which people can make those all-important emotional connections. And talk about emotional connection: when I told Dr. Gold about some of the stories I was receiving for *The Healing Project*, her eyes actually welled up with tears. It's amazing to find a doctor so empathetic and connected with her patients.

When the day of the surgery arrived, the hardest moment of the whole ordeal was when I had to leave Denise behind at the door of the operating room. But Doctor Swistel actually came out and walked me to the operating room. What a blessing. He even called me from his vacation later to check up on how I was doing.

I had a second operation after the first failed to clear the margins of my cancer, then sixteen weeks of chemotherapy every two weeks followed by radiation, every day, for seven weeks. I lost my hair in the first three weeks. I didn't want to wait for it to come out in clumps until it was all gone, so I went out and had it shaved. And with the reality of the disease giving me a yardstick to measure my priorities, I felt fine about having it shaved. It gave me another task I could do for myself, rather than just sitting around and waiting. Staying as active, and as proactive, as possible was very important to me. Throughout the ordeal I didn't stop working and went about my life with as much zeal as my varying energies would allow.

Following radiation, Dr. Gold told me that my biomarkers indicated I was a candidate for the new drug Herceptin which targets Her-2 and which had shown remarkable success in patients with aggressive breast cancer. Since the first round of chemo had caused damage to my heart and heart damage is also a possible side effect of Herceptin, I needed to be monitored during the treatments. If good things come in threes, my cardiologist, Doctor Allison Spatz, was my third miraculous doctor. She paid close attention to my case, and when she went off my insurance plan in the middle of my treatments, she actually refused to take payment for her work! I ultimately took Herceptin for a year with good results.

During chemotherapy, Dr. Gold also encouraged my interest in exploring alternative and complementary treatment, including herbal mixtures and vitamin supplements. This combination with traditional medicine did indeed help me. I know some people don't believe in the holistic approach, but for me I want to believe it worked. My immune system was pumped up when it should have been down, and I didn't get the flu like so many other people in New York that season. To me, that's an important point about dealing with cancer: it comes down to what you choose to believe. There are so many people with so many opinions and there are so many variables to consider. Ultimately, you have to do what's right for yourself, realize that you're not as alone as you might feel, and seek out the people who know best what it's like to be you.

And those are the people I want to help me build *The Healing Project* community. In addition to my daily work during my treatments and during my second round of chemotherapy, I began to develop *The Healing Project* as a place where people can contribute funds for research, time for connecting with and mentoring others and, most of all, a place to share their stories. Since then, *The Healing Project* has been collecting stories by those touched by breast cancer and other diseases for books like this one: books that inspire and inform for the road ahead and impart a sense of community for those caught up in dealing with the moment. When you're sick or afraid, it's a godsend to know that there are others who understand. These books are meant to be a companion for patients, their friends, and families, an oasis where they can find strength in shared experiences.

In addition to the books, we're also working on other initiatives through *The Healing Project,* including the Companion Network®, a "virtual support group" which will allow patients, family, and friends to connect with others in real time. I don't want anyone to have to feel the way I did that day of my diagnosis when I was walking through the city alone and afraid. There's so much strength in others—you just have to find them. I think of the people who were here for me: Denise, Doctor Gold, Doctor Swistel, and Doctor Spatz, and I realize how fortunate I was to have people who were willing to give of themselves and their time. The healing begins with giving to others.

So *The Healing Project* is part of my own healing, a signpost on my road ahead. And looking ahead, friends ask me if I consider myself cancer free. I choose not to. "The Big C" gives me something tangible with which I can measure my life. I guess I can't help being an entrepreneur, so I see the experience of cancer as an opportunity, with its own list of "Big C's":

To show Courage in the face of so much challenge.

To accept Caring as it comes.

To take Comfort from others.

To know it is OK to Complain.

To stay Connected with those you love.

To share with the Community your smiles, tears and fears.

To be Constant in your ability to rise above but never feel guilty when you can't.

To build Character for when you come out on the other side.

To Create kinship with others not as lucky as you.

To say I Can.

To say I Cannot.

To opt for Plan "C" if you must.

To take Control of your diagnosis and become your own advocate.

To believe in a Cure, if only for your heart.

To make Choices that you can live or die with.

Finally, with cancer you have to be ready to chart a new Course, for the rest of your life, no matter what the outcome. And it helps to see that others are busy charting their own courses along with you. That's what these stories are all about. Reading these amazing contributions to the *Voices Of* series convinces me that I don't really have a uniquely remarkable story at all.

The truth is *everyone* does.

Debra LaChance is the creator and founder of The Healing Project.

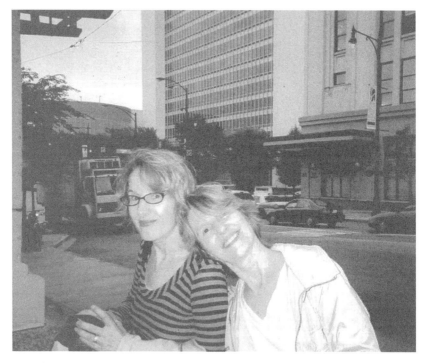

Denise and Debra LaChance

The Healing Project

Individuals diagnosed with life threatening or chronic, debilitating illnesses face countless physical, emotional, psychological, social, spiritual, and financial challenges during their treatment and throughout their lives. Emotional and social support from family members, friends, and the community at large is essential to their successful recovery and their quality of life; access to accurate and current information about their illnesses enables patients and their caretakers to make informed decisions about treatment and post-treatment care. Founded in 2005 by Debra LaChance, *The Healing Project* is dedicated to promoting the health and well being of these individuals, developing resources to enhance their quality of life, and supporting the family members and friends who care for them. *The Healing Project* creates ways in which individuals can share their stories while providing access to current information about their illnesses. For more information about *The Healing Project* and its programs, please visit our website: www.thehealingproject .org.

Research Hits Home
Michael S. Wolfe, Ph.D.

Over ten years ago, I began working on Alzheimer's Disease. My colleagues and I went on to make important discoveries about the molecular basis of the disease, with implications for new therapeutics. These discoveries eventually brought me to Harvard, elicited international speaking engagements, and earned me a reputation as a leader in the field. Nevertheless, I seemed to be virtually the only person who did not personally know someone with the disease. And with 4.5 million Americans afflicted with Alzheimer's, including almost half of all people over age 85, the chances of not knowing at least one person with the disease was quite slim.

All that changed during the past year. My own father, at the relatively young age of 65, began to voice concerns about memory problems. A former police officer in New Jersey who took early retirement and moved to Florida, my father loved to tease me about the warm, sunny climate he enjoyed while I weathered the winters of New England. Finally away from the harsh winters and his difficult and often dangerous job in the Newark area, Dad was free to play softball and golf to his heart's content. For a while, I dismissed his concerns about his memory: we all forget where we put the car keys from time to time, but as we get older we tend to read more into these momentary lapses than is justified. Living in a retirement community and having a son working on Alzheimer's also may have overly sensitized him, I thought. He was still quite a young guy, and the odds of him having a real problem were extremely low. In fact, at his age the chances were only about 1 in 100.

During the course of our lives, our bodies, especially our brains, produce a small protein byproduct called amyloid. As we get older, we are less able to clear out this byproduct, and it builds up to toxic levels in the brain, disrupting the connections between nerve cells that we need to think clearly and process memories. My colleagues and I discovered one of the enzymes responsible for producing this toxic byproduct and have been working to understand this enzyme better. Such understanding should help in the development of agents to block this process. Indeed, two agents that target this enzyme are now being tested in humans for their ability to slow or stop the progression of Alzheimer's. The hope is that such agents will lower amyloid and prevent Alzheimer's in a manner similar to how cholesterol-lowering drugs prevent cardio-vascular disease.

At some point during our weekly phone conversations, I realized that Dad did have a real problem and should consult with medical experts. As a Ph.D. chemist, I did not qualify, and anyway could not assess my own father's situation objectively. A year ago, he went to the Mayo Clinic in Jacksonville where he underwent a series of tests for his memory and attention. He was diagnosed with mild cognitive impairment, typically the prelude to Alzheimer's. Indeed, he was prescribed medication that I knew was for Alzheimer patients.

It was hard to say whether this medication was helping, although at least it did not seem to be hurting. The current medications for Alzheimer's have limited benefits. Although they stimulate the critical connections between brain cells and can lead to clearer thinking, they do little or nothing to stop the underlying problem: the inexorable loss of these connections and the brain cells themselves. I was well familiar with the limitations of these drugs, this being my primary motivation for working on the problem in the lab. How frustrating it was (and is), having dedicated my career to solving this problem but not being able to help my father.

His difficulties have become more serious during the past year, prompting a follow-up visit to the Mayo Clinic this past July. I flew down to Florida to accompany him on the trip. In many ways, this was a wonderful visit. We had more conversations in the span of three days than I could ever recall having before, probably because we never had this much time alone together. We also played chess, one of our father-son things to do over the years. In spite of his problems, he played a competitive game, which I found encouraging. We also had a few chances to throw a softball together, gradually ramping up the speed to challenge each other, just like old times.

But the trip was bittersweet. I watched him struggle with the one memory test I was allowed to sit in on. The neurologist gave the sobering diagnosis: very mild dementia, probable Alzheimer's. And his recommendations for certain lifestyle changes (driving, paying bills, having someone check daily about his medications) brought the point home that this problem was only going to be getting worse, that we should be planning accordingly. I had the surreal feeling of watching our own lives as if in a movie. This couldn't really be happening...it's too soon and too fast. Our work in my lab and other labs around the world had not yet advanced to the point where something could be done. Now the point of the research we were doing had clearly hit home.

We are in a position where, given the funds and the commitment, we can eventually prevent and treat Alzheimer's. How soon that happens will depend on the level of support and the depth of the commitment.

In the meantime though, I can still do something for Dad: I can be there for him, accept where he is now, and help him adjust to the changes that will be occurring in the coming years. After reading the stories in this book by others who have gone through this experience, I am encouraged that we can indeed make the most of what we have, where we are. This is not a movie. It's real life, and we must accept it and even embrace it as much as possible. One day, one moment at a time.

Dr. Wolfe is Associate Professor of Neurology at Brigham and Women's Hospital, a teaching affiliate of Harvard Medical School where his work has focused on understanding the molecular basis of Alzheimer's Disease and identifying effective therapeutic strategies. In January 2006 he founded the Laboratory for Experimental Alzheimer Drugs at Harvard Medical School, which is dedicated to developing promising molecules into drugs for the treatment of Alzheimer's Disease.

No Kidding

Charles E. McGhee

No kidding. I've been told I have Alzheimer's. That's a disease. I've been trying to remember if I have ever had a disease before. I'm 72 as I write this. Two years ago, Norma Jean, my wife, asked me if I would talk to our family doctor about my memory lapses. That resulted in a referral to a psychiatrist, who did a few cognitive tests and asked me a few simple questions like what time it was and what day of the month it was. He concluded a probable diagnosis of mild Alzheimer's. I remember my mother telling me I had had scarlet fever as a child. I remember having my tonsils removed. That was no fun. I've had my share of flu, diarrhea and the itch. But these are not real diseases; each is more of a nuisance. Alzheimer's, now that's a real disease!

After that doctor's visit, I went home and did internet searches on Alzheimer's Disease. I've always been a student. I studied engineering before entering the Air Force. I was trained as a flight simulator technician and served four years, but I really wanted to earn my bachelor's degree. I met the sweetest girl on earth during my first deployment. We were married within eleven weeks, just before the Air Force sent me to Morocco. For eighteen months we planned our life long distance. My wife supported my decision to leave the service and complete my degree, even though it meant changing her career dream to become a nurse. I always felt like we both earned that bachelor's degree. I have been a student ever since. I like to learn and this is why I had to find out about this disease.

Alzheimer's cannot be definitively diagnosed without an autopsy. That means the doctors are guessing. At the time, 2004, the literature estimated a diagnosis accuracy of fifty percent. That meant that I had a one in two chance that the doctor was wrong! I told the doctor this and offered to wager with him that he had made a bad diagnosis. He wouldn't take me up on it. (Smart, because how could I lose a bet like that?)

Now, two years later, more educated and sort of convinced that I do have the disease, I'm working on keeping what I've got, regardless. At the family gathering on the Christmas after the diagnosis, I told Norma Jean I wanted the children to know the diagnosis. Not the grandchildren; some of them would be too young to understand. I felt we needed the children's support, and it was only fair that they be part of what was to come. Norma Jean needed to get used to the idea of being a caretaker. I had to learn to make her role as easy as possible. It's been a little bumpy. But we have piloted this ship for fifty-one years together, and we can learn to bring this ship to a safe and peaceful landing.

Now, a year after telling the kids, life is good. We're getting a lot of wonderful support from them. I am enjoying badgering the doctors by telling them it's Tuesday, May 18th, 2006 before they ask me. Oops! I just looked at my calendar and May 18th, 2006 is not on a Tuesday. Oh, well! Life goes on...

After serving in the United States Air Force, the writer worked in electronics engineering before entering a career in the ministry. He was nearly seventy when he was diagnosed with Alzheimer's.

Acknowledgments

This book would not have been possible had it not been for the selfless dedication of many, many people giving freely of their valuable time and expertise. We'd particularly like to thank Amy Shore, Barbara Jeanne Fischer , Richard Day Gore, Ann Marr and A.B.C. Whipple for their work in reviewing all of the countless stories we received and for their editing prowess; Larry Bennett for steering the ship early on; Lisa LaChance for her assistance with almost every aspect of the project; Theresa Russell for her unending efforts to reach out to the many people and organizations making so many contributions to this book; Justin Cho for volunteering his time and focusing on all the details; Melissa Marr for her astounding, ground-up organizational ability; Drs. Marie Torroella Carney and Michael S. Wolfe for lending their extraordinary medical and scientific expertise; David Shenk for his interest and support; Victor Starsia, for setting the bar high and making sure we all made it over; and to the many, many people who submitted stories to us, for their courage, their generosity and their humanity.

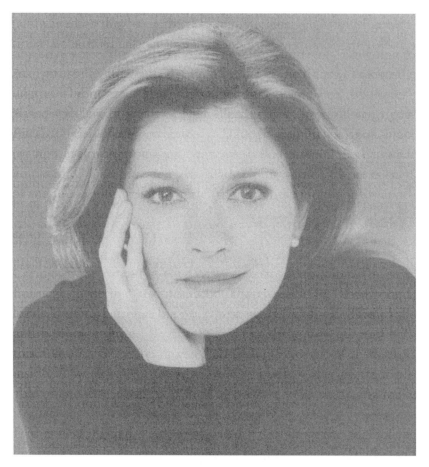

Kate Mulgrew, page 41

Photographer: Charles William Bush

Part I
THE PARENTS

Being a grownup means assuming responsibility for yourself, for your children, and—here's the big curve—for your parents.

—*Wendy Wasserstein*

Mothering Mother

Carol O'Dell

Letter to Self

Dear Carol,

So far, you've been taking care of your mother for a year and a half. You've stuck it out through crazy times, angry times, tender times, through hospital visits and home health visits and while everyone else comes and goes, you've stayed. You haven't had a vacation and no more than two days away this whole time.

I know you: I know that when your mother dies, you're going to feel guilty. You're going to think that you should have been kinder, not in a rush, that you should have done more with her, taken her more places, insisted the kids be nicer. I know you're going to miss her and wish that a million things had been different.

I want you to know you did the best you could. You remained faithful. You grappled with every decision. You let her into your life and your home, you and your family did what most people wouldn't even have considered doing, much less done. People aren't perfect, and if they try to be, then they're not real. We're not supposed to get it all right. Remember, you had to balance this with being a wife and mother. It's only natural to want to move forward and be more interested in your children—in those who are living. That's how the human race survives.

Remember, her emotions were always on an ever-widening pendulum, and Alzheimer's took them to frightening heights and devastating lows. You learned as a child that you couldn't trust her with your heart, although you kept trying. It just wasn't ever possible. That's okay. You know she loved you. And you loved her.

So go...love your children. Love your husband. Live life. Learn and grow and help others. Let it go.

Remember all the kindnesses—how Phillip built her apartment and put up her pictures, whatnots and books, how you tried to make it as much like home as you could, even before you did your own home. Remember stopping just to buy Klondike Bars for her. Remember the hot washcloths and how good she said they felt. Remember kissing her goodnight on her forehead, holding hands in the car and how much she loved getting her toes done. Remember how much she made you laugh and cry and want to scream.

You always knew you were alive with her. Remember.

Letter to Mother

Dear Mother,

I never wanted it to turn out this way. You, lost in confusion; me, overwhelmed and not knowing how to reach you. When you moved in with us, I was naïve enough to envision us sitting by the river, me holding your hand, you nestled under a lap blanket, and the two of us sharing memories of my childhood and your childhood. Somewhere in this idyllic dream, you'd doze. I'd feel the pressure of your hand loosen and I'd know you were gone. I would kiss your forehead and whisper, "I love you," as you began your journey home.

A fairy tale, I know.

The reality is that I tiptoe into your room each morning and hold my breath, watching for the rise of your chest. Not that I want you to die; rather I fear that you have. Your life seems futile. Your days consist of not much more than a series of meaningless actions and reactions. Are you now more driven by instinct? Do hunger and thirst and a need to be covered up and warm rule you in your wordless world? Am I trying to decide if your life is more or less valuable than mine? Who am I to say? Does this sound cruel? I don't mean for it to.

I wake each morning to view the remnants of your destructive night. I pick up the nightstand, the telephone that is no longer plugged in. There's a mound of clothes on the end of your bed that you've taken off the hangers. More work for me. You've taken everything off. Your skin is as white as the whole milk you drink, your eyes remain closed, shunning this world.

I thought you'd be different. I thought I'd be different. I didn't expect this. I miss you. I miss what little we had. I miss your humor, your laughter. You still laugh sometimes....

Integrity is what you do when no one's looking. I wonder how I measure up. It's not that I do cruel things—it's that I don't seem to be able to relax, to sit down with you, talk, read the Bible to you. I'm scared so I just keep on my feet. I want to help you make a scrapbook, watch some old TV show, anything that brings you a bit of pleasure. But it's too late. Those things no longer mean anything to you. Each day passes and my family needs me, but you need me too. I want to write, go for a walk, clean out the refrigerator, take a bath, anything to avoid you.

I haven't put you in diapers yet. You wet everything, and yet at least you still try to use the potty chair. I just can't do that to you—or me. I'm afraid the diapers will give you permission to give up. I know that day is coming, and I'm helpless to stop it, just another step in your descending world.

I guess what I resent the most is the endlessness of the situation. It's easy to be kind, loving and caring when there's a cut-off date. Cancer often makes people valiant. Families rally around loved ones and last wishes get fulfilled; but this just seems to run into oblivion. I fear the possibility of years of your existence, staring off into space, randomly screaming while I perform the duties of diaper changes, sheet and night gown changes, wondering why.

I tell you I love you, especially at night. I try not to let a night go by without telling you. If you could hear me, understand me, step back to see this whole picture of our lives, I think you'd be proud of me, of us. We've made a good family. I love you still. I love that you loved me. I love that I had a mother.

Carol O'Dell's literary works have appeared in numerous magazines and anthologies including *Southern Revival Anthology*, *Margin Magazine*, *Atlanta Magazine*, *The Pisgah Review*, *Timber Creek Review*, and *AIM—America's Intercultural Magazine*. She teaches creative writing and speaks on writing, care giving and adoption issues. Carol's book, "*Mothering Mother: A Humorous and Heartbreaking Memoir*" will be released in April, 2007.

Big Dan

Danny Simmons

Big Dan was my father, and although several inches shorter than I am, he was a man whose shoes were hard to fill. He had a Master's Degree in history from Howard University, earned the hard way, a benefit of being a WWII vet. He never ever talked about the war, but he did talk about social justice. His degree was in African American studies, not really a program offered in those days; he developed the interest on his own during and after college. Our house, unlike those of my friends, was filled with books by African American scholars and Big Dan filled his sons with the knowledge he learned. He didn't stop his teaching with us; he also ran a neighborhood youth corps project in Harlem, where he taught our history to both the "disadvantaged kids" and the counselors.

He was a civil rights activist, protesting daily in New York and around the country the injustices blacks faced in everyday life in America. Picket lines, sit-ins, arrests and civil disobedience were his tools, and my brother Russell and I watched and participated in the actions that formed our lives and which became his legacy.

Several unpublished novels and scores of poems were in closets and on shelves at home. Big Dan would whip a poem on us in a minute. "Sit down boy, and listen to this one," he'd say, "It's called 'Black

Man Behind the Shades'." Poetry about who we were and who he was. His poem 'Legacy' said it all:

This much I leave behind –

three fine sons,

and a bottle of wine

I hope my sons are understood,

and my bottle of wine,

will be good.

I hope that when I am dead and gone,

the love I feel for them

will go on.

I hope that I am not misunderstood,

but a good bottle of wine,

gives life zest.

And my sons,

I hope,

will provide the rest!

When I turned fifteen we started fighting about revolution, drugs, my friends, the way I dressed, almost everything. I left his household when I was sixteen, after a battle royal at the front door on my way to school. Big Dan, the man I watched place his life on the line countless times for what he believed in, would not let me out of the house with an American Flag sewn to the seat of my pants, to be bused to school in an all-white neighborhood. Blows were exchanged. He lost a tooth and I lit out of the door with the flag half ripped off and dangling from my butt. I stayed gone for two days and when I finally came back home, I packed and moved in with my grandmother, who lived two miles and a world away.

Still, Big Dan got me through the hard times, paid for New York University, paid for lawyers when I got busted for drugs at school and made the visits upstate when my education was interrupted by my eighteen-month residency in a New York State correctional facility. He made that trip almost every week. He fought hard to get me back into NYU afterwards, and succeeded: he was teaching Black History at PACE University at the time and the dean of the NYU School of Social Work extended a professional courtesy (after much begging and pleading on my father's part) to Big Dan.

There are so very many instances of this man's impact on my life and his impact on the other two Simmons boys, both of whom grew to be famous beyond any of our wildest dreams. After our parents split, Dad raised Joey (rapper Reverend Run of Run-DMC) for the next few years on his own until he remarried, to Shirley Ann, the mother of my best friend, Chris.

"Raising A Son Alone"

I now have a softer view of you

It took courage to do what you wanted to

At fist I considered it unkind

But thanks for leaving the kid behind.

We have grown fonder of each other

Since I began the dual role as father and mother.

We talk to each other a great deal more

Than we did as father and son before.

We are concerned with each other's health

What we have found is more than wealth.

We have the text book relationship

The corner boys would call it, 'hip.'

One night when I had a strange nightmare

He was there to show me that he cared.

He can cook, and so can I

I like to broil – he likes to fry.

Every now and then we disagree

But no one's perfect – not even me.

Some young girl is going to get lucky on day

And take my number three son away.

I will take it in stride because I understand

Every girl wants a fine young man.

In the end, it was Shirley and Chris who would have to tell me how Big Dan was doing. It was in 1998 when Shirley told me that Dad was starting to forget things. They were living in Florida. The pace was a lot slower there, so she shuffled it off to age and his not being as active as he used to be. But in truth, the forgetting had begun. It showed its face in small things: thinking he had to do something he'd already done; going shopping and returning with the wrong items. He'd compensate, cover his tracks, and not let on or get angry about the confusion and forgetting. At the same time, his physical health took a turn for the worse. He'd begun to stiffen; arthritis along with inactivity put him on the sidelines. I began to notice how my daily call to him in Florida got passed off to Shirley after a few brief remarks by Dad. "Hey man, everything fine; talk to Shirley." Tests confirmed our fears. Big Dan had Alzheimer's.

Now came the scramble for the newest, the best, the folk medicines to ward off the coming plague. Dad and Shirley moved to Atlanta, to live with my best friend-turned-stepbrother, Chris, and his wife Rhonda. They created a basement apartment, where Dad began to retreat into his own world, made up of old westerns and calling for Shirley (loud) every five minutes. As the Alzheimer's worsened, Big Dan got surly and demanding. Coupled with the atrophy of his limbs, he retreated to his bed or the lounge chair, where Alan Ladd killed Jack Palance in "Shane," day in and day out. As Dad's world narrowed, so did the world of those around him. In that household everyone's primary function became taking care of Big Dan. Now his primary caregiver, Chris had to leave his job; Big Dan became a full time job for him. Russell paid Chris a salary, but no amount of money could match the care and love that Chris gave Dad. Chris had known my father since he and I were in the second grade together. He too had listened all those years to Big Dan's poetry and philosophy. Long before Big Dan and Shirley married, Chris had become our fourth brother.

Dad was at his best when out for a drive with Chris. That's when he remembered stuff: old friends, old stories, places he'd been, and every so often he'd surprise us with flashes of his old brilliance, his humor, his wit and his sarcasm. No longer able to walk, he was chauffeured about in a wheelchair, and got around the house very slowly with a walker. I think what hurt me the most about his condition was when his confusion became obvious and he would hide his embarrassment with anger and silence. He didn't want the world to know that he was failing and I didn't know how to let him know that it was all right. That we were all right. That we loved him and wouldn't let him go. I wanted him to know that he had done a fine job, had been a stand up man, a good father, husband and friend. It was hard finding those words because as his fear and anger increased, so did mine. I wanted to rage at the disease and I wanted to fix him. I wanted to hide and I wanted my daddy back to read me poetry and teach me how to be less selfish, more confident and a better man. But instead I settled for "Hey man, I'm doing fine."

It took a lot to confront this every day, even if only by phone. I'd breathe deep before I called, knowing that I'd only get the "Hey man, I'm fine" before he'd pass the phone to Shirley. Sometimes I would hear him wailing unintelligible sounds in the background, and I'd steal myself a memory—something he'd said in some fight we had, in some poem he wrote in an intimate moment—when all I needed to do to be in his presence was to think of those things he had given to me.

In late 2004 we made a family trip to Jamaica, West Indies. He seemed happy but mostly hid in silence. But his eyes shined. I cried and he smiled during that trip as I sat alone with Big Dan on the balcony of his room and we watched the ocean. We didn't say much but as I sat in his presence I felt so much like the little boy who held his hand while we walked the picket line together. Here sat a great man wrapped in silence, watching the waves turn back on themselves, and for some reason I became alright with where he was and didn't have to retreat into memories of who he had been.

Big Dan died on June 12, 2006. I read one of his poems at his funeral.

Danny Simmons is a renowned abstract-expressionist artist, poet and author (*Three Days as the Crow Flies*, Simon & Schuster, 2003), the owner of the Rush Arts Gallery, Manhattan and Corridor Gallery, Brooklyn and the co-founder of the Def Poetry Jam.

In 1995 Danny, along with brothers Joseph (of the iconic rap group Run DMC) and Russell, the founder of Def Jam Records, created the Rush Philanthropic Arts Foundation. RPAF is dedicated to giving disadvantaged urban youth exposure and access to the arts, and exhibition opportunities to underrepresented artists and artists of color. The Rush Community Grants Program, also co-founded by Danny, each year provides direct funding to over 70 nonprofit organizations that offer educational programs in the arts to New York City youth. Rush's mentoring programs, including Rush Kids, Clinton Hill Kids Visual Arts Mentorship Program and the Rush Impact Mentorship Initiative offer to young people personal testimony to the transformative power of creative expression.

The Stolen Goodbye

Kate Williams

As I put the hot oil treatment on my head, the smell envelopes me. I am transported back to my parents' bathroom and the bottle of Aramis cologne that sat by my father's sink. It is the same smell. I go and buy a bottle of Aramis. I put a dab on my father's red flannel shirt that I have kept all these years. I breathe in deeply, and I cry.

My father is dying. He is in the final stages of Alzheimer's Disease. During his last stay in the hospital, my older sister and I went to see him. We took turns in bouts of crying. Different things set us off. For her, it was the shock of seeing him looking so old and frail. It wasn't our father; it was an old man. The bruises on his hand were shades of red and purple and looked painful. His skin was paper thin, scaly like a reptile. He was unkempt; I think this is what bothered my sister the most. His normally short-clipped hair and groomed eyebrows were wild and frightening. His breath smelled horrendous—something our father never would have allowed. It was difficult to reconcile this man with the image we both had of our father.

When we arrived, he was clutching the hands of a nurse who had just moved him to a bedside chair. He would not let go. I offered him my own hands and he reluctantly relinquished the nurse's, grasping tightly to mine. I sat, awkward, hunched over, glad to be of some comfort to him. As my sister began to cry, I gave him her hands and retrieved a book of poetry I had brought. I read from Robert Frost and he visibly relaxed, sitting back in his chair. He tried to talk. It was as if he had marbles in his mouth. I thought he was trying to recite one of his favorites, *Stopping by Woods on a Snowy Evening*. But maybe that's just wishful thinking.

We eventually settled into our old way of talking, my sister and I. We bantered back and forth, reciting poems that he had forced us to memorize as children, with him trying to pipe in. We were provoking some response from him but I couldn't tell whether it was in real time or simply vestiges of his former self, firings in his brain. When he tried to speak, signs of frustration would pass over his face. That's what killed me. The furrowed brow, the strain to put together words and make his mouth work properly. It was so hard to watch him struggle to speak.

We stayed for hours, bouts of conversation followed by long silences. But the silence was strangely comforting. He seemed relaxed and peaceful for a time; just our presence there seemed to be enough. His wife bustled in after her dinner date with friends, the atmosphere significantly altered. It was time for us to go.

And so I remember our visit now. I never know when it will come back to me. A smell. A phrase overheard from some other man from his generation. A song. A poem. A book. College football season. I am already mourning him and he is still alive. But he is just a shell of his former self. That is what Alzheimer's does. I don't consider this the long goodbye: I never got to say goodbye. It is the stolen goodbye.

Kate Ryan Williams was born in Houston and raised on a farm in Schulenburg, Texas. A fifth generation Texan, she is a graduate of Texas A&M University and the University of Texas. She has studied primates in Venezuela, worked for an Alaskan native tribe in Prince William

Sound and has been a grant writer for a national estuary program in Texas. She lives on the Texas coast with her husband and three sons. Her column, "Longest Days, Shortest Years" is published monthly in the Port Aransas South Jetty.

Language of Loss

Marjorie Carlson Davis

My mother was a talker, and she loved to entertain. My childhood bedroom adjoined the living room, and many nights I lay awake while my parents hosted parties. I heard my mother monopolizing the conversation, interrupting people and sharing long, detailed sagas I swear she'd told a hundred times before, usually embarrassing stories about my sister or me, like the time we ran away in our nightgowns. Her voice was loud, and to me, grating. *Does she have to tell that one again? She's boring everyone*, I'd think, my hands clenched by my sides. *Can't she just be quiet?* I took her behavior personally, as if her garrulousness reflected on me. I heard my mother talk and talk and talk and I was mortified.

Sometime in her late fifties my mother began losing words. I'd married and moved away by then, but back for visits, I would notice her struggle to speak. Such a change from the woman I knew. She'd use the wrong word for the one she wanted: fan for pan; walk a book instead of read a book. Sometimes her sentences would be a string of mismatched words or key words would be missing. Other times her voice would trail off in silence and frustration, a passage full of ellipses. My father, sister, and I would make excuses for her. She's tired, we'd rationalize. She had too much to drink at dinner.

But then other things began to slip, things at which this take-charge woman had been skilled: computing mistakes in the check book, an inability to plan. Simpler things, like confusion over which button to push on an elevator. She'd been an excellent cook, who could create a gourmet meal without using a cookbook, but now she told my sister and me that she'd lost her recipes. "Mom," we responded, "you never kept recipes. You'd just create meals as you went along." Her stunned and frightened expression communicated more effectively than words.

With no more excuses or explanations, my father took her to the Mayo Clinic. Maybe she'd had a minor stroke or the medication she was prescribed after her hip surgery had caused temporary memory loss. On the way back, they stopped for a quick visit with me in Iowa. I'll never forget the moment when my mother and I were alone in the hotel room, and she looked at me, her forehead drawn. "They think it's Al...Alz..." and her voice faded away. I had no desire to complete that sentence for her. I just wrapped my arms around her and held on, feeling the most extreme helplessness and panic I'd ever experienced, the way I imagine tsunami victims feel as their loved ones are swept away. Alzheimer's. No cure. An insidious thief, the disease that steals a person's essence.

My mother's decline was slow and steady and terrible: aphasia, dementia, even Parkinson's-like symptoms—tremors and difficulty walking. A woman who had always kept busy, taken charge and thought of others first, she retained her basic nature as long as she could. She worried about my father and was thankful when he met her increasing confusion with grace and humor. When she could no longer cook, she still wanted to help by making a salad or doing other simple tasks. Once she'd lost the ability to weave or knit—her creative outlet—my father would find her among her shoes with all the laces pulled out, as if she thought, somehow, she was still working with the yarns she loved.

In the first few years after her diagnosis, she'd still try to talk. I'd walk past her, wearing a brightly colored vest, and her trembling hand would rise. "I like...pretty..."

"You like my vest? Thank you, Mom." Or sometimes she'd just say, "You," her way of expressing recognition or love.

Eventually, words disappeared and my mother became mute, her expression wooden, eyes blank. Before she died, I would visit her and chatter about things I'd been doing or what the kids were involved with. I wanted to stay connected, and there was always the chance that she understood more than we knew. Yet I usually found myself lapsing into silence, helplessly stroking her hand or sniffing back tears. I'd never been a talker, and as much as I wanted to fill the quiet, to let my mother know I was there, I felt silly babbling on to someone who couldn't respond. I knew that if she were the one visiting an Alzheimer's patient, she'd have had plenty to say.

Sitting with her in the sterile nursing home room, I eventually realized something about my mother that I had not been aware of growing up. During my parent's parties, while I fumed about my loud-mouthed mother, I didn't hear the other voices or the laughter. I didn't realize then that she'd been the life of the party, transforming a roomful of awkward people, unfamiliar with each other, into a lively social gathering. How ironic that the first pieces of my mother stolen by the disease were the gifts I'd never acknowledged she had: her ability to put people at ease with her words and her skill at filling awkward silences with stories.

One comfort remains: my memory of the stories she'd told to our guests, the stories that once made me grind my teeth in embarrassment. One oft-repeated tale was how as a four year old, I stubbornly refused to demonstrate to her that I could count until she bribed me with ten pennies and a chance to play outside with the big kids. Immediately, I counted those pennies into my little fingers and skipped outside.

Today, I can still hear her narrating the penny story, complete with an emphasis on my perfect counting "...eight, nine, ten." What I hear now that I didn't during my childhood and teen years was her pride in my intelligence and independence...and her love.

Marjorie Carlson Davis is a writing consultant and freelance writer who lives with her husband, two sons and two dogs in Iowa City, Iowa. Her essays and fiction have appeared in many publications, including *Conscious Choice, Indianapolis Monthly, The Writer, Many Mountains Moving, Frontiers: A Journal of Women's Studies,* and the anthologies *Stories From Where We Live: The Great Lakes* and *Vacations: The Good, The Bad, and the Ugly.* She is currently working on a young adult novel.

Between the Synapses

Eileen Key

"Get this garbage to the curb tonight," she ordered. They pick up early, before you wake up." Mother jammed a paper towel into the trash barrel.

"Yes, ma'am," I pulled the bin toward the back door.

"Put your shoes on. You can't go outside barefooted."

I ignored the comment and continued trudging.

"Where are your shoes? Didn't I say put on shoes?"

The shrill accusation split my eardrums. I considered screaming back, but what good would it do? We played this game every Monday and Thursday night, fifty-two weeks a year. My mother had come to live with me, and the battle for dominion over the household raged. She often won, since I abhor confrontation.

"Use the slippers by the back door. Don't step outside without them."

A sudden bubble of anger shoved up from my tightened stomach, into my throat, and escaped my lips. "Shut up!" I said.

Stunned, we both stared at each other. I'd never been rude to my mother; it dishonored her. But there it was, bouncing on the airwaves between us. A roar of gut-wrenching words. A pounding from inside my brain which had escaped through my clenched teeth. A vital, necessary warning: shut up.

"I'm sorry, Mother…" I began.

"Well, who do you think you are?" She turned and huffed off to her bedroom, leaving me holding the trash, barefooted. Guilt surged through me. I considered chasing after her and apologizing again. Then I realized I was alone in the garage. Alone. Just me and the trash. In my bare feet.

I was over fifty, and if I wanted to walk on glass barefooted, I should be able to make that decision! Where did the fine line fall between honoring my mother and allowing her to rule my household? Her comments to my children often targeted their imperfections. In my desire to care for my elderly mother, was I sacrificing their self-esteem? I was getting crushed between the needs of two generations. Alzheimer's gripped the cells of Mother's brain. Bit by bit synapses were failing. Concurrently, my reactions intensified. How would we manage this rocky road together?

I limped, tender-footed, to the curb and leaned the trash can against it. A sudden urge to wail washed over me. Lifting my face to the stars, I cried out, "Father, what do I do?" Part of my heart wanted to hear from my dead dad, part of me wanted a heavenly touch. I waited; the pungent aroma from the trash can mingled with the night breeze. Was this the sum total of my existence? Where does my happiness, my life come in? I had single handedly raised three children and now was parenting again. Unfair, I dared to cry. Unfair!

I recalled the startled look in Mother's glassy eyes as she recoiled from my anger. Unfair. Her loss of life and memory outweighed my loss to the nth degree. Why should I complain: at least I had memories of what we had for dinner.

The silence continued. I waited. No one is guaranteed time. This was my time. This was my life now. Be content.

My heart's anger had surged and now subsided. Would this be the last time? I doubted it. Two people living in the same home would always have friction. Alzheimer's may cause more sparks, but God would be my damper. I smiled at the stars, walked to the house, and wiped my bare toes on the doormat. My feet stung.

Learning to live with this "new" mother has been a challenge. Alzheimer's Disease is progressive and irreversible. Simple forget-fulness is not a sign of Alzheimer's. It is more than just misplacing the remote control. Patterns of behavior emerge. Mother couldn't recall the most recent events, whether she'd eaten or who called on the phone. Slips in her speech, a loss of a word became more frequent.

When it became obvious her lack of memory was more than just normal aging, we met with our family doctor. He referred us to a neurologist. Using a few simple memory tests and her history, the doctor gathered enough data for a diagnosis. He prescribed the cognitive memory drug, Aricept®.

I noted a significant difference in her behavior when she began drug therapy. We ran out of the Aricept for two weeks, and I could see the confusion return. She was more agitated and forgetful. When we resumed the medication, she calmed down. Neither of these drugs caused an improvement in her memory, but they have slowed the progression of the disease.

Learning to live with someone who has Alzheimer's is a challenge. Several key factors help the care giver cope. First, accept that things will not improve. The parent, the spouse you once knew has been invaded by an alien force. Take time to assess this infor-mation and grieve, then move on. Dwelling on what *was* is not healthy. At this point, you must accept the situation and learn to deal with it.

With my teenage children, this meant teaching them about their grandmother. I wanted them to honor her and understand how different she had become. But the now is their reality, the woman they know: harsh, confused, scared, full of conflicting emotions. We walk a fine line at times, but love prevails. Their impatience has waned as they've learned about the disease. A multi-generational household can work.

Arm yourself with the facts. Find books in the library, talk to the doctor. The Internet abounds with information. The Alzheimer's Association has a variety of booklets, which they will send you. Avail yourself of these resources.

Often, it is important to connect with other care givers in this unique situation. Find local support groups online or in the phone book. Many local organizations even have daycare services where you might take your parent or spouse while you are busy with an errand or appointment.

Caring for the patient in your home requires adaptation. The environment must be "user-friendly" for the elderly. Throw rugs, cords, any impediment for walking must be removed. Safety rails and bath aids should be installed. Often locks on bath and bedroom doors need to be reversed so patients can't lock themselves inside. A wealth of information and "how-to" articles are available online listing common steps to prepare your home and make it safe.

The most difficult preparation for a care giver is mental. Parenting your parent is especially difficult, since the reversal of roles is unnatural. My bare feet didn't bother me, but it triggered the mothering instinct in my mom. She'd cared for me for decades and she remembered that. Arguing or debating any issue with an Alzheimer's patient is fruitless. They no longer have the capacity to reason. Learn early on to acquiesce. It's no longer a fair fight— you lose. You have control of the situation, of course, but the verbal battle over any issue goes to the patient.

Maintain a sense of humor. If you have a good friend or family member who will support you, laugh about some of the incidents in your life. Laughter is good for the soul and cleanses many black moments.

Be flexible. Time doesn't move at the same pace in the patient's life any longer. What used to be a five-minute ride to the beauty shop now seems like a long trip for Mother. Outside of our immediate home environment, the world is a frightening, fast-paced whirl. She is unable to operate the way she did. Remember, they *can't* remember. It is aggravating to repeat yourself over and over, but they have been robbed of the ability to process the data given to them, to have it remain on their hard drive. Drop the phrase "Remember I just said..." from your vocabulary.

Take care of your physical, emotional and spiritual needs. There is help available. Check with the local agencies to see if your parent or spouse qualifies for home services. Ask another family member or a friend to sit with them. Carve out some time for yourself. Do not let the disease swallow your life, or you'll be of no use to the patient.

The war against my mother's brain still rages. I ignore many of the words of advice and I give in to my frustration sometimes. But there is underlying love and peace. What I've been given in this care giving experience far outweighs the daily irritations, despite having to wear shoes.

A retired teacher, Eileen is now a freelance author and editor. She lives in Texas near her three children and two grandchildren.

The Treasure in Care Giving
Marie Ellen Alberti Galasso

There I was, alone in the ocean in the middle of the night. Darkness surrounded me. I feared that the sea would swallow me up, but I knew I had to get to shore. I looked around frantically to see if there were any other option, but there was only one: I had to wade through the crashing waves, water up to my neck, until I reached land. Feelings of fear and doubt that I could make it to the other side of that vast ocean consumed me; yet I had no choice but to forge ahead. When I awoke, I had to gather my senses to assure myself that it was, indeed, a dream.

I never saw it coming, really—oh, yes, I saw my parents slowing down some. I noticed my mother becoming a bit more forgetful and perhaps I even noticed she might call me in the afternoon and talk as though we had not just spoken that very morning. Still it all seemed to happen so suddenly. I remember the doctor explaining to my dad and me that my mother's CT scan confirmed a number of TIAs, or mini-strokes, which she'd had throughout the years. In a short time, she was diagnosed with dementia, and, little by little, I saw my mother become physically and mentally weaker. I watched my dad care for her as well as he could. I tried to be there when it was just too much for him to handle. At times I felt exactly as I had in my dream—I wondered if I would make it to the other side. At times I was exhausted. I wanted other family members to help more; I wanted to grab hold of a life preserver. But much of the time I felt as though I were drowning.

It's been a number of years since then, and there is much I learned from the experience. So much of it I wouldn't trade or change for one moment: talks with my dad about his love for my mother, reminiscing about past family events, simply placing my hand on my mother's face, enjoying the feeling of her soft skin against mine, tender words shared with loved ones as we recognized the brevity of life. We learn to slow down in the midst of the storm, to enjoy the tender moments, to realize that reaching out for help is not a sign of weakness but of wisdom. In ways, the experience refined my character, as I slowly became a person with the capacity to be patient, compassionate, and insightful. I learned to love someone enough to be there even when it wasn't pleasant, loving her enough to accept her weaknesses and her strengths, to be able to forgive her for past mistakes and to be able to look at my own mistakes and let them go.

Too often we forget to think about this aspect of care giving. Similar to giving birth and raising our children, this is the most challenging work we've ever undertaken, but the experience enriches us beyond words. We might need to reach out for help; we might need to talk to someone about it all; we might cry at times and wonder if we can do it any more. All of these things are true for sure, but the caregiver is also the one who is there when he or she is needed most, and for that very reason the bond of love grows deep and wide. For that very reason we grow, change, and, yes, eventually swim to the safety of the shore.

Not only have I experienced care giving personally, but I have had the privilege of meeting many care givers through the program I coordinate. I have learned so much from them. Many have expressed appreciation for a place to meet other care givers in support groups or for the counseling they receive to support their new roles. They learned a great deal about their own family backgrounds and how it affected their care giver relationships. Many have found that understanding themselves and their own reactions better has given them strength they didn't have before. Others have learned to step back, learning the difference between responding and reacting. Many have learned the importance of setting boundaries and have come to recognize that placing a priority on their own needs is crucial if they are to continue in healthy care giving relationships.

Dr. Bernard Lown has written, "Only a relationship bonded by understanding and respect can deepen into a true healing partnership." We can find the pearl in the midst of the sand, the beauty in the midst of our circumstances, and, if we are fortunate enough to find that treasure in care giving, we have come closer to the heart of who we are, and we are changed.

Marie Ellen Alberti Galasso, LMSW has served as the Care Giver Program Coordinator of Services Now for Adult Persons, Inc. (SNAP) since 2003. She received her Master of Social Work Degree with a concentration in Aging and Health from Hunter College School of Social Work and is currently serving on the New York City Family Care Giver Coalition.

It Isn't the End of the World

Barbara Jeanne Fisher

I remember as a little girl falling down on the pavement and scraping my knee. Although it was a minor hurt, at the time it seemed major to me. I began to cry and when I was certain I had my mother's complete attention, I cried even harder. I will never forget how much better it felt when Mama washed my knee and applied medication and a bandage. She kissed my cheek, held me close, and whispered, "Honey, I know how much it hurts, but believe me, it's not the end of the world."

Years later, when I was engaged to be married, my mother tried to encourage me to take time and be certain I had found the right person for a lifetime partner. I was head over heels in love and chose to ignore my mother's warnings. After all, what could a mother know about such things? Later, when my significant other turned out to be a real rat, my heart was crushed. I didn't think I could possibly go on living. Even though she had never approved of the relationship, Mom never said, "I told you so!" Instead she just held me close, and let me cry. Then sharing my sadness, as only a mother could, she told me, "I truly know how much you are hurting, but, believe it or not, this isn't the end of the world."

She was so right. Only a year later I met my husband, and a short time after that we married. In the next six years, God blessed us with five beautiful children. I had never felt as loved or so happy. Then, just when life seemed almost too perfect, I was diagnosed with multiple sclerosis. I was devastated, and certain my life was over. When Mom came to the hospital to see me, I could see she too had been crying. She sat on my bed, and for the longest time we just held each other, unable to talk. There just didn't seem to be any right words at such a wrong time. Finally, with tear-filled eyes, Mom took my hand in hers and said those same words again: "I know this is a terrible, difficult time for all of us to accept. We have to put our trust and life in God's hands now more than ever. It could be worse, you know. As bad as it seems, it isn't the end of the world."

Indeed it wasn't. For the next twenty-one years I lived a very fulfilling and rewarding life. I not only lived to see my five children grow up, but also my five beautiful grandchildren. In spite of my illness, my life had been truly blessed.

Then a year ago, my mom was diagnosed with Alzheimer's. Before she progressed to helplessness, she had temporary periods of normalcy. During one of these times, while talking with me, Mom asked, "Now, what is this disease I have? What's wrong with my head? Please, please be honest with me!"

She listened carefully as I tried to tactfully explain her expected prognosis the best I could. I felt like a traitor, imposing a terrible life sentence on someone who had always been there for me. Because she was a very intelligent person, I couldn't imagine how painful it was, being told of her mind-stripping illness. My heart was broken, I wanted to run away. As I spoke, she listened so carefully, grasping my every word. For the longest time she remained quiet, lost in a world of her own, seemingly so far away. Then suddenly her eyes met mine. It was so like my Mom, even in the midst of her own private hell, to put my feelings first.

"Now why are *you* crying? *I'm* the one who is sick this time. You must be brave for both of us. Oh, God, I know how much this hurts you, but regardless of what happens to me, you've got to be strong. In spite of what you think right now, I promise you, this isn't the end of the world."

Her disease progressed rapidly. On rare occasions Mama would smile, but most of the time she was extremely depressed. Many of her friends and relatives stopped going to see her because it made them feel uncomfortable. She was no longer able to hold me close, say all the right things to soothe my pain. She couldn't assure me, in troubled times, that my world would continue. I so missed her gentle encouragement, but I knew that it was my turn to be the strength in her life. Because she no longer remembered the words, I said for her what she taught me so long ago. Mama still understood kisses, and returning the ones she gave me for so many years helped her.

Three days ago my brother, sister and I stood crying in my mother's room shortly after she passed away, wondering how we would go on without her. It was time to say goodbye. None of us were ready, but we had no choice. As I stood there, a sudden peacefulness touched my heart, and somewhere from a far away place, I could hear my mother whisper, "Cry for the loss that you feel in your heart, but also be happy for me, for I am with God in a place that you can't begin to imagine. I am so happy now. Yes, honey, I am gone from your life, but never from your heart. For the last time I promise you, *it isn't the end of your world.*"

Barbara is a prolific writer whose stories have been published in numerous magazines. She has eleven stories appearing in the *Chicken Soup for the Soul* books and has published four children's books. In her first novel, *Stolen Moments*, many of the emotions portrayed by the characters come from her experience in dealing with illness in her own life. She is the owner of the Open Book Store in Fremont, Ohio.

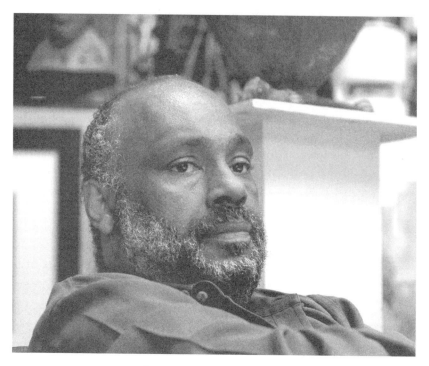

Danny Simmons, page 7

Dancing Shoes

Marguerite R. Greenfield

This Thanksgiving we were at Kay's new condo, and we ate off plates on our laps, cranberry sliding into turkey and mounds of potatoes restraining a cascade of peas. Our informal perching replaced the long mahogany table in the now empty house in Westchester where our parents had presided over the clatter of cutlery, laughter and anxious young mothers quieting impatient children. The year after Dad died we had fled for the holiday to the beach to avoid the empty seat at the head of the table, huddling in mournful celebration at a country inn. This time, loss prompted a retreat to the city, and we welcomed the familiar confusion of a holiday dinner. We had spent too many hours in the delicate dances of "oh no, you take it," as we cleaned out, then sold the family house. But there was no empty chair at this feast. Mom was with us. The empty place this time was where she used to store our names.

"Well! Look who's here!" she exclaimed when she arrived. "It's … all of you," she faltered, her face clouding, but she recovered quickly in the scrum of greetings and hugs.

"I'm Margo," I said as I took her coat.

"I know, dear," she said. I watched her as she walked into the room, her thin frame as erect as ever, but her clothes hanging a little looser and her eyebrows penciled too dark. She smiled and cocked her head at each of us in turn. "How lovely to see you," she said. "Where are you living now?"

John settled her into the deep wing chair and went to get her a drink. Her smile faded as she gazed worriedly at the scurrying grandchildren. I picked up the old leather photo album off the bookcase and sat next to her, opening to the curling black and white snapshots glued to its stiff black pages.

"Which one is you?" I asked. Mom brightened and pointed at a solemn-faced girl in button shoes posed against a marble pedestal, and another of her standing next to a dapper man holding a straw boater and a cane. "And that's my father." She said. "I was the oldest." She paused. "He's gone now, isn't he?" She looked at me uncertainly, her brow furrowing. I nodded and changed the subject.

"Where is the one of your graduation?" I asked. She turned the page and pointed to a young woman in cap and gown standing behind a "Class of '38" banner.

"I was class secretary," she said proudly. She turned a few more pages of photographs of long ago holidays, pausing at a formal shot of her parents posed before a fireplace, their children arranged around them. She closed the book and held it to her chest, stroking the smooth leather.

A few minutes later, John tapped his knife against his glass and led the toasts, ending as we always did.

"To Charlie."

"To Dad," we echoed. Mom looked up, waving her empty glass.

"To Dad," she repeated.

"No, Mom," my sister Liz said gently, "to our dad—your husband. To Charlie."

"Charlie?" she repeated, her brow furrowing, "Where is he?" My sister Kay moved quickly. "Hey, someone needs a refill!" she said. She topped up Mom's glass and the awkward silence was soon filled with the sounds of clattering plates, laughter and squealing grandchildren, of the familiar family feast. As the meal wound down, Mom's smile grew a little vague and she leaned back in her chair, her eyes unfocused, her wig a little crooked, struggling to stay attentive when someone asked her a question or passed her a plate. She watched my sister and brother across the room waving their hands in familiar disputation, her head pivoting back and forth as she tried to follow the talk of elections, candidates and war over the intermittent waves of cheers rolling out from the television in the den.

"Why are you whispering?" she said, suddenly angry. "It's rude. If you want to talk privately, you should do it somewhere else." She had forgotten that she was hard of hearing. She put down her coffee and pulled herself up. "It's already dark. Where's your father?" she asked anxiously. "We need to be getting home. I hate it when he keeps me waiting like this." We had learned to let these moments pass. She paused for a moment then looked up blankly. "Where did I park the car?"

"It's okay, Mom," Kay said. We're on it." Her voice was soothing. She curled her arm around Mom's thin shoulders and walked her to the front hall. Physical movement was an easy distraction. "We're going for a walk first. Bill's going to bring you home when we get back." "Home" for Mom was now a residence, with familiar furniture but strangers in the hallways and unfamiliar food.

"Home. I can't remember where that is," she said, turning to me, her shoulders sagging. "Oh, I've gotten so stupid!" She switched gears like this a lot. Anger. Fear. Confusion. Shame. "Aren't we going to have dinner?"

"We'll eat when we get back," Kay assured her, helping her into her coat and waving insistently at her husband. John poked the kids and they crowded into the hall, grabbing hats and jackets.

"We'll come along later," Liz said, turning back towards the den. "The boys are watching the game." Uncertain, Mom turned back.

"They'll catch up to us," Kay assured her, taking Mom's arm and raising her eyebrows at me. I slipped over to Liz, whispering, "We agreed to this. Kay made this plan and already paid the deposit; let's just do it."

"Madame?" John turned to my mother, extending his elbow and bowing slightly. "May I escort you?" My mother nodded grandly, and they sailed out the door.

"Bowling?" I had asked doubtfully when Kay had suggested it a few weeks ago. Who'd want the flashing lights, clattering balls and loud music after a holiday dinner?

"Well, we can't take a walk in the country," she had replied. "And after a while, nine of us crowded into the apartment will be pretty claustrophobic. The lanes are only three blocks away. They have a bar and great music. C'mon, it'll be fun."

"You're insane," Liz observed. "She's 82 years old. She doesn't know how to bowl." "Well, you're the one who says she should have more exercise," Kay replied.

When we got to the lanes, Bill started explaining the rules. John made sure everyone had a drink and Dan pulled out a paperback and slipped into a corner of the booth. The kids were arguing over the choices on the jukebox. Liz reached to tie Mom's bowling shoes. Mom looked down at the grimy striped shoes with disgust and swatted Liz's hand away.

"I'm not wearing someone else's shoes. Look at them; they're so ugly." Katie was filling out the score sheet and grinned at her grandmother. "Come on, Grandma, you can't play without shoes; if you don't hurry, I'll take your turn."

"Oh no you won't," she retorted, and leaned backward to let Liz tie the laces. She pushed herself up and let Kay lead her to the ball rack. As Kay bent to choose a ball, Mom stood at the head of the lane, a little dazed by the flashing lights, the roar of balls flying down the lanes and the crash of flying pins.

"Look how lost she is! This isn't a good idea," Liz muttered. "I can't bear to watch this." "Maybe it'll fire up her competitive instincts," I shrugged, though I was worried that she'd drop the ball on her foot and for the next six months be asking why it hurt. Kay passed Mom the ball and tried to help thread her fingers into the three holes. Mom kept pulling away.

"I can do it," she objected, trying to balance the ball on her arm while pushing a thumb from each hand into the grip.

"No, just one hand, Mom...not your forefinger...there, you've got it. Now, line up your thumb with the row of pins, drop your arm, swing it back and roll the ball down the lane."

Kay tried to position her arm, but Mom shrugged her away. She took three strides to the foul line then stopped. Dropping her arm, she swung the ball back, then forward, and then dropped it onto the floor at her feet. It bounced twice, then wobbled down the lane a few feet before sliding into the gutter.

"Damn it," she exclaimed as the ball rolled desultorily down the trough and the mechanical arm lifted the pins. She stamped her foot and turned back toward the bench. "This is a stupid game."

"Wait, Mom, you get a second chance," Kay called and walked her back to the rack where the balls lurched up with a pneumatic hiss.

"Hey Mom," Bill called from the next lane. "Do it like this." They both watched his effortless three-step approach: the coiled arm, the backswing, the snap of his release. Their eyes followed the swift course of the ball and listened to the crack as four pins went flying. He smiled happily then turned back to his brothers-in-law and called for another round of beers.

Kay picked up the ball, and again Mom struggled with the grip.

"I've got it," she said, irritated. Again she lifted the ball, walked the three steps, and stopped at the head of the lane. Carefully lowering the ball, the weight of it pulling on her thin frame, she let it go with another hard bounce on the polished floor. The manager's head came up; I was afraid he was going to ask us to stop. This time, the ball kept rolling.

"There you go, Mom," Kay called out. "You're getting the hang of it."

"Atta way!" Bill called.

"Oh my God, it's still going!" Liz laughed as the ball ambled on.

"I think I can, I think I can," Katie began to chant, and Liz and Frank chimed in. Players at the other lanes began to look over. Mom lifted her head. She straightened her shoulders and lifted her chin. The ball approached the wedge of pins and gave a gentle push, slightly off the center. Two pins wobbled, then tilted towards the others, and in a slow motion, clattering cascade, laid waste to the remaining eight. Lights flashed and the sound system bugled a celebratory trill. Children and grandchildren hollered hoorays and a few players at adjoining lanes added their applause. "Good job," I murmured to Kay as we clapped in delight. Mom bowed at her audience.

"Smile, Grandma!" Katie called out, and snapped a picture.

We watched as she shimmied a little victory boogie, pumping her arms and pirouetting on the toes of her ugly green shoes. I had watched her waltz at weddings and envied her grace then. I had never seen her dance a jig. She bowed and stepped off the stage in the rushing pleasure of the upturned smiling faces of people who knew and loved her. Radiant, she had forgotten that she didn't remember our names.

Margo Greenfield is a lawyer who lives in New Jersey.

Caught in the Net

Kate Mulgrew

We should be grateful, I know. It wasn't cancer or MS or a crip-
pling stroke. It was nothing more than the Disease of the Decade,
catching yet another fish in its wide, deep net and dragging it
slowly under water, down into a vast and mysterious world of
plaques and tangles, where one becomes easily lost until spat out
on some distant shore, unrecognized and unrecognizable. A pecu-
liar washing up, replete with soothing sounds from the mouths of
caregivers, who say quite amazing things like, "She wasn't a bit
belligerent, you know. She just got sweeter and sweeter. See? Isn't
she a darling?"

To me, she looks frozen and far from sweet. In fact, to me she
looks downright dazed and if I peer at her long enough, I will
guess at little shards of horror glinting in the far recesses of what
was once her mind. The caregivers and certain others smile as she
accepts the spoonful of mashed egg; they laugh out loud when she
smacks her lips and puts her napkin over her head.

Down, down, deep under the water she goes. When first caught in
the net, her lungs were mighty organs and she fought hard not to
lose her breath, not to lose her way. She took me into her bedroom
and asked me to help her find a way out that would not leave her
brain in gooey, tar-like tatters where one and all could approach

her as if she were a rather good-looking, mentally challenged girl of ten and shout, bizarrely, "'How are you doing today?" Oh, how she resisted the very shadow of the grotesque joke she was about to know intimately. She did not want to be seen getting into the tub with her socks on, she did not want her oldest daughter to strap on rubber gloves and clear her excruciating bowel blockage. She did not want to fall seriously and hauntingly in love with her youngest son, she did not want to fill the pan with turpentine and put it to boil on the stove, she did not want her car keys forced from her hand, her underpants replaced with diapers, her food cut into infantile pieces, her precious books left like orphans on the windowsill.

She wanted out before Out took over. But I could not assist her in this, her final cogent request, because I am a creature of reason and I still clung to her with the madness that reason bestows upon hope.

So down she went, and we all came tumbling after.

The children of this woman do not like this Disease of the Decade; it sets them adrift in strange waters full of hostility, jealousy, , and fury and unplugged, unending grief. They fight over the last vestige of her normalcy, each one sure that his or her name will be the last one uttered by those beloved lips. They watch as she falls down, then they help her into a wheelchair and, finally, someone just puts her to bed.

She is brought little trays of tempting morsels she has long since ceased understanding or caring for. And she is thirsty, and this will last a long, long time, even as she stares the blank, hungry stare of the forgotten, and looks into the eyes of one of those she once loved deeply. And the one she once loved receives this emptiness as a mute prayer of longing and despair.

The day arrives when the thirst abates and she closes her mouth to what is left of nourishment. And all of her chicks come to roost and to watch and to count each and every breath the drowning woman must take before it is over. It takes five days, so powerful is the heart of this slip of a woman, who bore eight children, buried two of them and searched all her life for the mother who perished in childbirth. This same small, rather delicate woman had violent, outsize feelings, soarings and dippings of passion, bright red gashes of sorrow, her gifts that took possession early and later became mountains that she scaled with trepidation and delight and something like great courage.

The Disease of the Decade, otherwise known as Alzheimer's Disease, as popular, well known and trend setting as it is, would not have been my first choice. It would have been far better if she had taken an accidental bullet, or stumbled into the path of an oncoming train, or stood with her arms outstretched to the sea and dived in, of her own volition. Whenever she took me to the airport, she would say, "Something catches in my throat when I have to leave you. I really cannot bear prolonged good-byes." Then she would turn on her heel and be out the door, you see, in a flash.

Kate Mulgrew first became known to television audiences as Mary Ryan on the daytime soap opera *Ryan's Hope*. She has played a range of characters in several television series and miniseries, most notably *Kate Loves a Mystery* (also known as *Mrs. Columbo*). From 1995 to 2001 Kate played the role of Captain Kathryn Janeway on *Star Trek: Voyager*—the first woman to play the lead role in any of the popular Star Trek series. Her impressive stage career includes appearances at the American Shakespeare Festival, the O'Neill Festival, and at the Mark Taper Forum in Los Angeles. She toured for several years in *Tea at Five*, a one-woman show in which she portrays Katharine Hepburn. Kate is a member of the Alzheimer's Association National Advisory Board.

Assessment Number Two

Maryann Lesert

Gina, Lou and I are sitting at the kitchen table, having coffee. Dad is outside, puttering around the shed. It's a very windy spring day. Lou and I had arrived to tell Dad that someone named Fran was coming over to do a "senior health assessment," Gina, sounding winded, greeted us in the driveway. "Your Dad's out back trying to get himself blown away along with the shed."

We walked to the cleared-out garage. Dad walked in, pointing at us with his middle finger, as he's always done. "Good, good. You're here to help. That door," he said, "the wind just took it and *wham*!"

He went to his workbench, fumbling with a spread of tools: a wrench, some washers, an assortment of screwdrivers and nails. But he couldn't find the hammer—I figured Gina had hidden it from him. I watched Dad pick up and set down tool after tool, as if wanting his hands to tell him which one was right. "He didn't set the hook on the door, and it got blown open too hard," Gina told us.

The last time I visited, Dad was trying to fix the sprinklers, which, for some reason, meant he had to cut the hose to the water heater. Now Dad found a handsaw. "Oh no-ho-ho, don't you take that out there," Gina scolded. "Come on. Come and have coffee. The girls are here."

In the kitchen, as Gina warmed the morning coffee in the microwave, Dad stood, glancing out the window, shifting his weight from foot to foot as he often did when fixated on something and wanting to get to it. I put my hands on his shoulders and told him the wind was too strong to work outside. But as soon as the coffee was poured and he couldn't figure out where to sit, he was out the back door. Gina hollered after him, too tired to chase him, "Lee, don't you dare nail anything on that shed!"

The three of us talk now, preparing for questions Dad will be asked about eating, dressing, and showering. He's been struggling with shirts, doing odd things with the sleeves as he tries to put them on. Sweatshirts, Gina says, work best.

Curious to see what Dad is doing, I get up from the table and go to the window.

I should be helping, as Lou tries to elicit the response we need from Gina about when she wants us to move him but I stand, fascinated, watching Dad try to "fix" the shed. He's holding a piece of molding in his hands, trying to make it fit in some magic, matching place. It's not the complete lack of his spatial awareness that fascinates me, but rather the mystery of what must be going on in his mind as he stands before the open doorway of the shed, unable to decipher the spaces and shapes before him. First he places the thin strip of wood across the opening on a diagonal. The molding doesn't reach to the other side. He toddles to one corner of the shed and holds the strip of wood flush to its edge. When that doesn't work, he moves to the other side of the shed and puts the board flush with that corner. I watch as he repeatedly slides it up and down. But the board is too short, so he reaches overhead and places the board under the roof line, extending it downward towards the open doorway. What is happening in his mind when he does these things?

"You guys ought to come and see this, how he's trying to make the molding fit," I say. Lou and Gina stare back at me, blankly, wondering how I can find this interesting. "I know," I say, "but it's fascinating, in a way, watching as he tries to fit the shape." Gina looks tired. Lou looks at me with one eyebrow raised, beaming *shut up* into my eyes.

Dad is trying to place the molding parallel to the angle of the roof now. Only instead of tucking the board up under the roof slant, he positions the board diagonally across the opening. But the double-door opening is too wide.

I want Gina and Lou to see what I see. Gina just smiles tiredly at Dad's antics and my sense of wonder. Lou's eyes are telling me to be more sensitive to how exasperating it is for Gina to live with a man with whom she once traveled the world, but who is now in her backyard trying to fit a piece of molding in all sorts of wildly impossible positions on the shed. But I can't attend to their need for camaraderie. I can only watch. So I apologize. "I know it's sad. I do. But I can't help it. It's so interesting to watch the process."

"I'm sure it is," Lou says, eyeing me hard, "when you don't spend every waking minute with the person."

I try to narrate what Dad is doing, but Lou and Gina ignore me, talking to each other about the upcoming health assessment. Gina isn't ready to talk "assisted living" with Dad. "Not quite yet," she says, so for now we're telling him that these in-home visits which Lou and I have arranged are standard for seniors like Dad, to see if he might benefit from services such as an emergency call box or meals on wheels.

Last week's assessment with Shelley, the Director of Care of our second-choice assisted living facility, did not go well. With French-manicured nails and a frilly V-neck dress, she didn't look like any nurses I know. Shelley asked Dad direct questions: "How do you do with dressing yourself? Any problems with buttons or shoes?"

Dad grew quiet, sitting with his hands clasped in his lap, nodding and smiling uncomfortably. Shelley wrote in codes, "AE30" and "I-15" in boxes on a preprinted form. Later, when Lou made me call and ask Shelley what assessment form she was using, Shelley said it came from "property management."

Lou is pressing Gina for answers now. "Gina," Lou says, in her objective voice, the one that means *she's organizing,* "I'm going to ask you something directly and I want you to answer honestly, whatever you feel." Lou is younger than I am, but this look—along with hands out before her, directing, mouth set—says to me *Back off, I'm handling it.* She was Daddy's girl. "If we find a place for him, we're assuming you want us to do this soon. Is that what you want?" I keep my eyes on Dad. He's returned to the corners of the shed, shifting left then right, placing the molding flush with one corner, then the other. But he keeps coming back to a faded shape along the right edge of the doorway.

"If he wants it," Gina answers.

Lou sighs. "Let me rephrase that. That wasn't fair." Lou sounds legal. That's what bugs me. But these are difficult words, and she hates confrontation. "Okay, how soon do you want us to do this?"

Gina hesitates, her "ho-ho-ho" barely audible as a break in her breath. "I don't know (ho-ho)...I don't want to hurt him."

Dad is back to that shadow of faded paint along the edge of the doorway, which represents where the piece of wood in Dad's hand had fitted to the shed. Dad is sliding the molding up and down, parallel to the ground, when it needs to be perpendicular.

A year ago, we were disturbed by his "visions." I borrowed his car to drive to a workshop in Louisville last spring, and he called me several times to warn me about a leak in one of the hoses. By the time he'd called a fourth and fifth time, I envisioned a Medusa of hoses being unleashed from under the hood. "They'll come right out and pop your hood," he told me. "And the oil. You just can't believe the oil. They'll get to spraying it so thick, hoses every-where, just a-thrashing, and you can't see a thing." Then there was the respiratory virus he caught over the winter. He'd tell us how his lungs were just "slap, slap, slapping" against his chest when he coughed, and sometimes, one of his lungs would "slap right out his back with the waterfall." Gina decided, finally, that she could not care for him any longer when he woke her up in the middle of the night and said, "Gina... I forgot how to go to the bathroom."

Lou is telling Gina about Fran, the director of our first-choice assisted living facility, who is due any minute. Fran's nails, she said, are short and she has the hands of a nurse: well-used, often-washed, and slightly red. When we visited Fran's facility and asked questions about licensing and staff ratios and training, she smiled and understood. "It's like trying to find good childcare, isn't it," she said. Fran is a degreed registered nurse. Shelley, with her polished nails (forgive me), is a licensed practical nurse. An LPN directing care?

I'm trying to leave Gina and Lou to their more serious talk. I think Dad is about to get it. He's back to that strip of faded paint along the edge of the doorway, and he's placed the molding upright, nearby. A few slides and he'll have it.

"Hah! I think he's got it."

Gina must have already seen this played out a hundred times, because she stands up, moves to the window, slides it open and hollers. "Lee! It doesn't belong there! It belongs on the door!"

She grumbles as she sits. "It's got to go on the door, it's the inside piece that fits on the door."

Thankfully, Dad doesn't have the door. I stand and watch as Dad, distracted, holds the molding on an angle again, and moves toward open space.

I want to "shush" Gina. *Redirect, never correct,* as Fran would say. He almost had it. But my eyes fill with tears, and I decide to be thankful. Gina is exhausted, and I should be happy to have these moments to watch, so I apologize. "I'm sorry."

"I know," she smiles, "I know, Hon." And with that Gina is up again, rising from the chair and reaching out to widen the open casement window in one motion, as if she's done this so many times that it is an automatic, physical reaction to her sense of frustration. "Lee! Get in here and have coffee with your daughters!"

Gina is living minute by minute with the mechanics of Dad's memory loss. A year ago, we sat in a specialist's office, amazed that Dad could no longer tell time or draw a box or sign his name. Now she's living with a man she accompanies more as a "sitter" than a girlfriend. Dad has lived with Gina for ten years, here in this house where Gina had already taken care of one dying man, her husband of four decades, before she and Dad gave each other rings but decided not to go through a marriage ceremony and all the legalities. Gina can't do it all again. Dad's doctor, in our most recent consultation, called Gina Dad's "umbilical cord". But he warned us that Gina's blood pressure, with her lack of sleep and all the anxiety, was reaching dangerously high levels. It was time for Gina to care for herself.

Back inside, Dad stands away from the table with his coffee cup. He looks young still, even at seventy-six. His dark hair is graying, and he's bald on top, but he has been for years. Up until this year, he was still playing "old-guy" softball. Sure, his teammates had to correct his stance at the plate and remind him which base to run to and when to put his glove on, but he was out there, enjoying the game. This year, the coach asked Gina not to sign him up. Now he cannot be left alone, not for a minute, it seems. He is waking up in the middle of the night, telling Gina he wants to go home.

Dad turns to go outside, but something about the dining room window catches his eye, and he moves toward it. The casing is open farther than the sliding storm window, which, just moments ago, Gina pulled back so she could lean out and wave him in; I can tell he doesn't like the relationship between these shapes. Can't something fit? He tinkers with the heavy wooden casing and the inner storm window, sliding them back and forth. It's just like one of the social workers said, "There's no sense in correcting them when they get fixated on something, they're trying to find closure."

As I watch Dad strive for some success with shapes, I can't stop feeling there's a map to it, a particular puzzle or pathway for each person; I can see Dad's. He's always been a fix-it person. Always. And when there were no standards or models to follow, he made up his own—like the homemade sheet metal monster of a snow sled he made that we called the Blue Whale, the one that trapped us under its weight when it capsized on the edge of a snow bank and our legs flailed for the new home movie camera as Mom, behind the lens, laughed until she cried. Or the new floorboards Dad soldered and bolted under the driver's seat of Lou's rusting old Nova. I get goose bumps watching him, thinking that for everyone, and for Dad, too, there must be some neural pathway that misfires and reroutes in ways that correlate to how that person used their brain all along. And I wish, so fiercely sometimes, that we had more time to slow down and watch and to listen. To take note. In so many ways, I wish we simply had more time.

But Fran is coming; Fran with the hands of a nurse. Fran and her facility, with four wide-open wings and wardrobe closets with white linings—no hallways or dark closets. But Fran's facility doesn't have showers in the rooms. Dad would have to make his way to the end of his wing, carrying a drawstring clothing bag. And soon, they may not let him shower on his own. But this is a silly detail to get hung up on, isn't it?

Dad has been waiting; I can feel it, for me to look at him, that same gradual awareness I used to feel when the kids were small and they'd shuffle and stare and wait for me to notice them. He catches my eye and he points, with his middle finger, toward the window. *There*, he communicates with a huge, triangular smile. Hah-hah! *There. I got it.* After much tinkering, he has positioned the window casing and the inner screen so that they line up exactly. Exactly.

There. I say to myself, nodding in his direction. *There.* For now, one piece fits.

The author's award-winning plays include *The Music in the Mess*, *Samhain* and *Natural Causes*, a finalist for the Princess Grace Foundation's National Playwright's fellowship. Her first novel, *Base Ten*, was written while she earned a Masters in Fine Arts in Fiction from Spalding University. This story is an excerpt from her current novel-in-progress, a work that draws upon her real-life experiences with her father's Alzheimer's Disease. She lives in Michigan.

Mary's Life, Mary's Death

Aaron Liebowitz

It was a quiet death on a late winter afternoon. Her final moment of life followed hours of labored breathing under a morphine induced sleep. With her final breath her pale green eyes opened one last time. It was over. On March 3, 2005 Mom died.

It was not a wrenching moment. It was very quiet. Her two sons were with her in the silence of her solitary room in the nursing home. My brother and I looked at each other with nothing really to say. We gave each other a hug and said goodbye to this 88 year old lady who had conceived us and birthed us and fed us and continued to mother us through the haze of dementia caused by Alzheimer's Disease—and she did so right up until her final days.

My experience with my mother through her years of decline may not be like others whose relatives are brought down by insidious protein amyloids wrapped around their brain cells. Mary never wandered away from home. She never became physically aggressive. Mary declined with the strength and courage with which she had lived her whole life.

Born in the years just before the "Great War," Mary lived in a family where grief and loss were all too familiar. Becky, the eldest daughter, died of Malaria in Mexico. Jackie, the elder son, and my mother's most beloved brother Sam both died of muscular dystrophy. Her sister Annie died of breast cancer. Then came the Great Depression, and the Second World War. By then my mother was married and had given birth to a stillborn son while Hymie, her young husband, fought the Nazi terror across the beaches of Normandy, following General Patton through France, Belgium, and Germany.

We were the proverbial "blue collar" family in the tenements of the Lower East Side of Manhattan, eventually moving out to the "country" setting of Queens County where we boys could be outside and ride bikes.

My mother's decline began decades after the death of my father. She lived those years alone in her cozy little apartment that she loved so dearly. When work as a saleslady in Manhattan was no longer possible, Mary sought paid and volunteer work with preschool children at the local community center. Her final volunteer assignment was, ironically, as a companion to the center's elderly Alzheimer's members.

Mary's dementia came on softly and quietly, like a kitten gently tiptoeing into a room not wanting to be seen. Forgetfulness, yes... but don't all older people begin to lose some memory? She could laugh at herself, and we could make her laugh, too. That's the magical thing about her dementia; she ultimately lost all of her memories, so everything was new and fresh to her. She couldn't remember her husband without seeing his picture. She sometimes called out for her mother, not remembering the long life she had lived since she was her mother's child. But she was always able to laugh when her sons or her sister Terry would visit. She laughed at what an awful cook she was. She laughed at the old world proverbs, sayings, and songs that she carried in her mind from the old country of her parents. She thought she looked young and beautiful in her wedding picture.

Mary was an avid walker. Before the arthritis, osteoporosis, and stenosis of the spine crippled her and made her frail, she would take walks of three, four, or five miles. When the dementia began, she wouldn't realize how far she had walked; often she was physically unable to get home. Mom didn't think twice about stopping someone, getting into a car, and simply asking if he or she was going her way. Inevitably, they were all going her way. What could only be described as a reckless disregard for safety on her part was universally met with kindness. Did they see her vulnerability and innocence? I think they did.

More than anything, Mary's dementia brought out her very best. In her healthy years, she needed to be feisty and strong, never allowing herself to be taken advantage of. In her dementia, she was softer, more open and kind. She often amazed herself with the acknowledgement of her age. Where had all those years gone? Yet, she always said that she felt, inside, no different than when she was a child. Mary loved dolls; the delight in her face if I brought her one was no different than my daughter's when I brought her a doll for a birthday.

Mary would need to go to the doctor regularly, and I would take her. Getting her in and out of the car became more and more time consuming and difficult. The real challenge, though, was sitting with her in the waiting room. There we would be, she in her wheel chair and I in the tufted leather seat. Around us sat the other patients waiting to be seen and the intrusive receptionist, who obviously didn't have enough to do.

"Are you married?" Mom would ask me. Immediately, I was the center of attention and the only entertainment for everyone there with nothing better to do than listen.

"No, Mom, I'm divorced."

"Ohhh, divorced. Who were you married to?"

"Her name was Jane."

"Did I know her?"

"Yes."

"Was she Jewish?"

"Yes."

"Did you have children?"

"Yes."

"What are their names?"

"Dana and Richard."

"Why did you get divorced?"

"Mom, this isn't the place to talk about this!"

"Why not? Tell me what happened."

"No, we're not talking about this now." Groans of disapproval would be heard from the "peanut gallery" assembled in the waiting room, now disappointed at my cutting off the inquisition.

"Look at your tie!" she'd continue. "How could you go out of the house like that?"

"What's the problem with my tie?"

"The two ends aren't lined up. Isn't there a loop to hold them together?"

Finally the receptionist would say "Mary, the doctor will see you now." Thank heaven. I'm saved! But as uncomfortable as she made me feel in public, I knew she still wanted to be my mom and for me to be her little boy. I miss that.

Before the fall that landed her in the hospital, the nursing home, and the grave, Mary reveled in coming to family gatherings for holidays and special occasions. She wanted to be noticed. Mary wanted very much to be at the heart of "family". She would sing songs and show us how she learned to use her hands when she took belly dancing lessons. She liked the expression that as the "matriarch" of our little family, she was the keystone of the building our family had become and we were the arch.

The course of our lives tracks like a bell curve. Our birth leads to a long period of development. After reaching the fullness of maturity, the curve begins its inevitable decline. From sharing the decline of my mom, I got to experience two important things. First, the latter portion of the bell curve of our life, in many ways, mirrors the earlier, ascending part of the curve. I saw Mom as the child her mother knew and the young wife looking beautiful in her wedding dress. The second, more profound experience was a lesson: she taught me what to expect in my own decline by her example. She taught me how to face, with power and dignity, what awaits me.

Aaron Liebowitz is the father of two, a social worker by training and the Executive Director of Adults and Children with Learning and Developmental Disabilities Inc., a not for profit organization serving some 3,000 people in Long Island, New York.

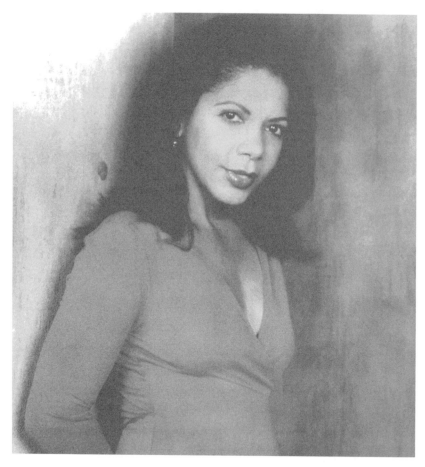

Penny Johnson Jerald, page 167

An Acquaintance

Marsha Kostura Schmidt

Rita Hayworth's eyes. That is what I remember most about the moment I first learned about Alzheimer's Disease. A small blurb in the paper, a daughter's announcement of the horrible news, accompanied by a photo. Gone was the long red hair, the voluptuous looking eyes, the temptress smile. The person staring out from the photograph was dressed in a trench coat, unkempt gray hair flowed wildly around her face. And the eyes, wild and uncontrolled, stared out like a frightened animal...

I pull into the parking lot of the assisted living facility on a crisp November morning. I am taking my mother to a doctor's appointment and I am running late, so I rush inside. The facility is a lot like a dorm. Each resident has a room with a kitchen area and a private bath. It does not have the acrid, antiseptic odor of a nursing home. There are common areas for activities and watching TV. A woman comes in to do the residents' hair once a week and a manicurist keeps everyone's nails polished. When my mother rails about being in a home, I tell her I'm jealous, since it's like being at a full service resort year round. She likes that idea.

The nurse's aide tells me that Mom is in the recreation room with the other residents for the morning chit chat. I find her sitting at a table with a half dozen of her neighbors. All but two of the residents are women, grey haired, some stooped with the hump of osteoporosis, others leaning on walkers, a few trailing an oxygen tank. My mother is 81. Her hair is dyed a honey blond and her skin is only slightly wrinkled, not reflecting her advanced years. She has shrunk a few inches with age, but she stands straight and can move well and the other residents often ask her for help. One of her neighbors likes to call on her to help her get up with her walker. My mother rolls her eyes but holds the walker still with her strong grip. The contrast with the other residents is so stark it is easy to wonder why my mother is there.

"Mary, look who's here," says the activity director, pointing at me. My mother turns. Her eyes have a glassy, almost wild look. She cocks her head and starts to giggle.

"Hello, mother," I say cheerfully. She is still studying me.

"Mary, do you know who this is?" the director asks. "It's your daughter." I sit down next to her. My mother laughs again. "Oh, is it you?"

"Which one am I?" I tease. "Let's see. You have Michele, Maryanne, Michael, Matthew and I'm ..." I pause, waiting for her to fill in the blank.

There is silence. The other women are waiting. The director touches my arm and whispers, "Tell her who you are."

"I'm Marsha, Mom. Remember?"

"Oh yes, I know you. You're Marsha." She draws back to get a good look at me. She doesn't seem convinced that she knows me or that I am the Marsha she remembers.

"We're going to the doctor's now. Are you ready?"

"I'm going with you?" She looks at the activity director for assurance.

"You go with her, Mary," the director says. "It's okay." She gets up and follows, but still eyes me with a bit of wariness. I take her to her room and help her into some warm clothes. I button her coat and find her gloves and scarf.

> *She had long, wavy, chestnut brown hair, a strong nose and full cheeks, much like Barbara Stanwyck. World War II called and she joined the army out of high school. It was a good time for her. From a mining town in the coal country of Pennsylvania, she went out into the world. A large box in the attic held her cherished mementos of that time: photos of army friends, notes from the boys overseas, and her uniform.*

It is an hour's drive to Pittsburgh, along a route we had traveled many times. In days past, the drive would have been filled with stories. She would share her memories about her life growing up, being in the Army, raising five kids. Sometimes we would talk about politics and world affairs. She always watched the news and was up on everything. On this ride, it is eerily quiet. She plays with her fingers, nervously rubbing her hands on her jacket. I try to start the conversation.

"So I just took a trip to Arkansas."

"Arkansas, Arkansas," she mutters, trying to think. "Have I ever been to Arkansas?"

I make an effort to help her remember. "Yes, you were stationed in Little Rock when you were in the Army, weren't you?"

"Little Rock, Little Rock," she ponders, those words searching for some memory. "Was I in the Army?"

"Yes, you were in the Army. Don't you remember?" As soon as I utter those words, I wish I could take them back. But I am floored. She has never forgotten the Army. For the past few years, she has talked about it incessantly. I try desperately to recreate her past for her. I explain to her who she used to be.

She was a strong woman, working most of her life to help my father run his dry cleaning business. She took care of the books and pressed and ironed and sewed the clothes. She raised five kids. She kept a garden and she could grow African violets from one simple leaf cutting. I can see her leaning on the sink, gazing out of the kitchen window over the fields, a cup of coffee in her hand, watching the sun rise, on the look-out for the family of pheasants that roosted behind the house. She fed them in the morning while the frost still powdered the grass. She would call me excitedly to report the addition of a new baby or another hen following the male.

"There are lots of things I don't remember," she says with some resignation. "I'm going crazy. I am going to be like one of those lunatics that I see on the first floor. They have them locked up. That's where I'm going to end up some day." She has watched several of her fellow residents make that trip. After one too many tantrums or one too many verbal or physical assaults on the nurse's aide, they disappear. Their room is emptied, and then readied for a new resident. My mother knows they have been taken downstairs to the Memory Care Unit.

I don't disagree with her, but it is hard for me when she has these moments of clarity, when she knows that something is not right with her. On the lucid days, she searches frantically in her mind for names and places, trying to prove to herself that she can remember if she tries. But she finds blank spaces, mixed up Picasso-like pictures of the past with parts gone missing. She sometimes pleads with me to not let her end up on the first floor. She once asked me if she could move to Belgium. When I asked why, she said, "Don't they let people die there?" She meant the Netherlands, where assisted suicide is legal.

More often she is lost. She doesn't remember her grandchildren although their photographs smile out from the wall. I once found her studying the photographs, trying to match names to faces. At other times she turns the pictures face down so she doesn't have to look at strangers. She was a tailor but she can't remember how to sew. She tells me she finds it hard to believe she could ever do anything like that. She always had a way with plants, but now her plants are faded and withered and she doesn't understand why.

When I think back, I can't remember much about my mother as part of my life. I was the youngest of five, and while my mother was there, she seems to fade into the background. But as adults, we became friends. She supported me and took delight in my life, listening to my tales of adventure and travels and encouraging me to live life as fully as I could.

The conversation has come to a standstill again. She points at a house. "I think I've been there before." I follow her finger but I know that she has not been to this house. I remind myself, whatever you do, do not argue with her. "Have you?" I say in the agreeable voice I would use on a six year old. I try another topic.

"What did you have for breakfast this morning?"

"Breakfast. Fssht. I don't know." My question was foolish. Time has no meaning for her. The morning has long since evaporated. We ride in silence.

"What do you do?" she asks politely. I explain. She asks for my husband's name. I tell her, knowing that she lights up when she sees him. I explain what he does for a living. She listens attentively. I wait for her to ask me again in a few minutes or a few hours.

Suddenly she starts to talk. The facts are jumbled. There was an incident at lunch. Two or three people involved. She talks about this girl or that man. She cannot remember names so there are none. The timeline is mixed up. I can't follow the story. But I nod in agreement and try to listen intently to find some path, some meaning in her words. She stops, satisfied that she has told her side of it. I try not to feel the crushing weight of my heart as it falls.

> *How many times have I wished I could forget something, just wipe it from my mind? Relationships I wished I hadn't had. Ugly things I wish I had never said. Embarrassing moments bubbling up out of the depths to remind me that I am less than perfect. But when I'm with my mother I know that what is passed, in ten years or in ten minutes, is what defines us. In layer upon layer of time, we find out who we are and who we might be. While I can hold my mother's memories for her, only she really knows what they meant and how they formed her self. We are not who we are if we do not know where we have been. We can have no ties to others or to ourselves without yesterday to weave the string.*

We have been driving in silence for some time. At a loss as to what to say, I fall back on the only topic left.

"Haven't we been having wonderful weather?"

Marsha Kostura Schmidt lives with her husband and cat in Silver Springs, Maryland. She is an attorney by profession, practicing in the field of American Indian law. She is an essayist and photographer whose work has been published in several newspapers and journals including *The Christian Science Monitor* and *The Washington Post*.

Once Upon a Memory

Carol Bogart

My father, a proud and frugal man who "never wanted to be a burden to his children," arrived at my door with my mother one fall day, looked down at my 2-year-old son, and asked, "Where did she get *him*?" Dad's forgetfulness had become a subject of much concern. Although a possible explanation was his bout with pneumonia a few years back, I was a journalist who'd done a fair amount of medical reporting and suspected something far more sinister.

The warning signs started before my son was born. Dad, ordinarily a "hale-fellow-well-met" type, became uncharacteristically suspicious of a young man mom hired to help with the mowing of their 43-acre farm. Maybe he saw this young man's help as evidence of his failing health, maybe it seemed like a harbinger of the loss of independence. Dad gave Mom a hard time whenever the young handyman showed up to mow or tinker with the lawn tractor. She'd been bewildered, hurt–and a little annoyed–the day he told her, "Maybe you should have married *him*." The helper was more than 40 years her junior. When Mom, then 76, shared the story with me, I listened with a growing sense of dread. "Mom," I said, "that's not normal."

Mowing the hills and tractor path to the back field had always been Dad's domain. For 30 years, he'd been industriously transforming the weedy abandoned mess we bought at auction in 1959. Our first year there, Dad cleared all the brambles from the hillsides, replacing them with 200 seedling Blue Spruce. The trees, he said, would grow tall and spread their soft needles on the ground, creating a habitat for deer and other woodland animals. Once, as we sat talking, Dad told me why he liked trees so much. He said it was because "they'll live on long after I'm gone."

When I left for college with no clear direction in mind, Dad said he thought I'd be good at broadcasting. It was one of the rare occasions I actually listened to either parent. Dad had always wanted to be a sports writer but didn't think it was practical, so instead he majored in business at Ohio State. Dad graduated when he was 28, got a job with "a future" and, after a five-year engagement, he married Mom. Within a year, my brother came along. The year, 1936, saw the country just emerging from the Great Depression. The little family scrimped and saved. Mom darned their socks, clipped coupons, made rag rugs and quilted comforters with my aunt and Gramma. Thirteen years after my brother was born, in 1949, the folks had me. We all lived in a little house across the street from the high school where Mom was the school librarian.

Dad was well-thought of at his job with an auto parts company that had its warehouse on Cleveland's Far East side. Each day, he commuted from home an hour or so each way and impressed his employer with his work ethic. Eventually, he was promoted to warehouse manager. Not long after my brother left for college, Dad was ready to strike out on his own, a bold move for a man who had just turned 52. He cashed out his company stock options, sold the little house in Olmsted Falls, and we all moved in with my mother's mother. For that first year, Dad struggled to get his first auto parts store off the ground. He was one of the first NAPA jobbers in the country.

Anxious to move Mom and me into our own house, he wanted the rural life he'd known growing up. Then Mom's sister told her she'd heard about a farm for sale on North River Road. She even found old photos of the two of them picnicking there as girls. Dad was the winning bidder for the farm. He paid $18,000. It was 1959.

Mom and Dad planted ornamental trees and flowering bushes. Dad spent hours and hours in his garden. After preparing the soil, he would stretch lengths of string to guide his seeding. As the plants came up, each row was laid out in a perfect grid, just so. Dad's garden produced an abundant crop of peas and strawberries, asparagus and green beans. A big red flag that something wasn't right with Dad was when he lost interest in his garden. That last year, Mom fired up the rototiller and said, 'C'mon, Lloyd, let's till a few rows." Dad shambled out and gave it a try. After just a row or two, he lost interest.

Mike, my son, was born in October, 1985. Dad saw him for the first time that Christmas when he and Mom came out to Denver. Even then there were signs. Mom and I bundled Mike up and took him over to the nearby park to push him on the baby swing but as we walked Mom said, "We mustn't be gone too long." Quizzically, I looked at her. "I wouldn't want your dad to wander off," she said, without further explanation. Her own father had been prone to "wandering" in his final years. This is no small thing, I thought. "Is something wrong, Mom?" I asked her.

"No," she said, "but maybe we should start back now."

I only lived a couple blocks away and we'd been gone less than half an hour. Yet when we opened the door to my apartment, there was no sign of Dad. The panic in Mom's eyes was unmistakable. We found him in the lobby, lost, confused, and miserable. He said he'd decided to come and find us, then didn't know which way we'd gone. When he tried to go back to the apartment, he couldn't remember which floor I lived on. Mom and I both made light of it as something that could happen to anyone, but I started to take note of how often Dad seemed to lose his train of thought and how often my mother's eyes would cloud with worry.

Within a year, Dad would forget I'd had a baby.

At home, Mom couldn't leave him for a minute. Dad had always enjoyed building a fire in the basement fireplace, but one afternoon, he propped a sheet of plywood in front of the blazing fire, evidently mistaking it for the screen. Mom, upstairs in the kitchen, smelled the smoke as the "screen" began to smolder.

She finally agreed with me that it was time for Dad to stop driving when her highway horror stories convinced me he would kill them both. Even at 80, he was still driving to each of his now-five NAPA stores scattered around northwest Ohio. He'd come home and tell Mom how some son-of-a-bitch semi drivers had scared the hell out of him when they passed him, blaring on their horns. Heaven only knows what *Dad* had been doing. I don't remember why Dad was in the hospital for a brief time about then–maybe it was his diabetes–but when he got home, Mom had squirreled away the car keys. For the most part, he forgot to ask about them.

One of Dad's business partners watched out for Dad as his memory failed, once picking up a $50 bill he'd left as a tip on his $9 lunch. The gift of a microwave made it easier for Mom to whip up something quick for them to eat. She told me she was glad she didn't have to use the burners on the stove. Depressed and scared as she was, her own concentration wasn't what it had been.

She finally gave up trying to take him to church. Getting him dressed took hours. She'd just have him ready to go, and he would disappear. Upstairs, she'd find him putting on a second, or even a third, shirt over the first one. Or, he'd taken everything off and gone back to bed. Asked how long she planned to try to manage by herself, Mom said simply, "As long as I can."

"Are you having any fun, Mom?" I'd ask. "Not much," was her wistful answer. Mom took her wedding vows seriously. She'd pledged to remain faithful "in sickness and in health."

"Mom," I begged her, "you don't know how many good years *you* have left. Don't you want to see Mike graduate from high school?" Balling up a resolute little fist, she punched the air. "College!" she said, sounding certain and determined.

I offered to move back home to help her, but she said no. Maybe she was afraid Dad's erratic behavior wouldn't be good for a little boy. Near the end, Dad was often irritable and unreasonable. He was also incontinent. Sometimes he'd forget to put on his diaper, and mom would spend a good portion of her day cleaning up accidents. Such a difference from the man she'd loved for most of her life, a man who never, ever failed to close the bathroom door. "He was always so modest... " she'd say, her voice etched with misery and exhaustion.

During one of their last visits to Denver, I was reading in my room as Michael napped. I heard a sound at my door and sat up. There stood my dad, a Depends adult diaper clutched in his hand. As I met his eyes, he said brokenly, "I guess I don't have very good control." Dad and I had had some very rough years as I was growing up. Mom always defended Dad, saying I'd "provoked" his angry outbursts. I suppose I did, but I didn't mean to. I yearned for the father I saw in photos holding aloft a chubby baby dressed in pink with a shock of coal black hair. I wanted him to love me, and was mad at him for years because I thought he didn't. Now, to see him standing there, so vulnerable, so humbled... I walked the few steps to him, held him and said, "You're a dear daddy, that's all I know."

I made arrangements for him to see geriatrics specialists in Denver, praying one of them could help him. He'd always been so articulate, so well-spoken, a great story teller. "You must be so frustrated," I said once when, again, he'd lost the thread of a story. Eyes downcast, shoulders slumping, he simply nodded. There were no answers, though. I watched hope die in my mother's eyes.

Still, she couldn't make herself put Dad in a nursing home. Mom had been a Red Cross volunteer "grey lady" who'd often visited the nursing home-bound elderly during my high school years. She couldn't bear to consign Dad to a fate she feared for both of them. Being his sole care taker, keeping him at home, was, she believed, her duty. And maybe, she thought, just maybe he'd get better. Seared in her memory, too, were my father's tears on the rare occasions she took him to a nursing home for a few days so she could spend a little time with Mike and me in Denver. Trying to bring him with her had become more than she could handle.

Ultimately, worry and hopelessness killed my mother. In an ironic twist of fate, viral pneumonia took Mom 11 months before Dad died. Grieving the death-by-inches going on inside Dad's ruined brain stripped Mom of her immune system and even, I think, her will to live.

In another irony, it seemed as though Dad's outlook improved once he moved into a nursing home for good. No one there had known him before. No faces looked anxious when he couldn't finish his sentences. No one gave "accidents" a second thought. Observing the home's other residents, Dad could see that at his age he still had reason to be grateful. Walking down the hall with him one day, we passed an ancient woman, her hair in long, faded braids, clutching a Raggedy Ann doll to her chest. Dad stopped and stared. Taking him gently by the elbow, I moved him along. "See, Dad," I said, "it could be worse."

He glanced at me and answered, "That's a fact."

He seemed to only dimly remember the loss of his wife, his farm, his pets. Once, though, when I called from Denver he asked, "Carol? Is your mother there with you?" And, at times, he seemed excruciatingly aware of his limitations. I told him what an autopsy of his brain would soon confirm. "You have Alzheimer's, Dad," I said. A look of pure relief washed over him. This wasn't his fault! He couldn't control it! He could stop blaming himself. At last.

I called my father every day and learned how to communicate with him as you would a child. A mother knows what her baby wants. A toddler only has to say a word or two and the intuitive parent reads his mind. I'd known my father for 40 years and had no trouble finishing sentences his impaired memory could not complete.

As the end approached, Mike, now 4, went with me to Ohio as one health crisis or another sent Dad to the hospital–five times in those last 11 months. I was thankful that Dad always knew him. He never failed to place a feeble hand on Mike's head, or draw him into his lap and smile, happy for the visit from his grandson.

In that last year, I made a point of soliciting my dad's opinions, his desires, his wise counsel. A few years earlier, when he'd had pneumonia, he'd said to me, thinking he was dying, "I hope you'll forget some things." I knew which painful things he meant. The yelling, the hurtful criticisms, the "being too busy" to do things with me, and even, sometimes, a lost temper that turned physical. Now here I was, not too many years later, driving an airport rental car across rural Ohio in the dead of night, my small son asleep in the back seat, thankful to have this last chance to heal old wounds, to know and love my dad.

The day I took Dad on one last trip to see the farm where he'd grown up, we drove through a McDonald's for a cheese Danish. I paid the bill and handed him a napkin. Dad watched the money change hands and said, "Wish I could help you." I took his hand–firm, warm and strong inside his leather glove.

"You've been helping me all my life, Dad," I said, and meant it.

A single parent, the author is a newspaper editor and columnist who worked for twelve years in TV news as an anchor/reporter. Her reporting has won or been nominated for four Emmy awards, a medal from the International Film and Television Festival of New York and multiple Associated Press awards.

Mom Had Alzheimer's

Ruth A. Brandwein

How does one start to talk about the disappearance of a mother? Not her physical disappearance, but the gradual disappearance of her personality, her personhood.

When it began, I went into denial. It was after my father died that my sister and I noticed changes in her behavior, but I, a professional social worker, attributed it to the depression that is common after the death of a lifetime companion. My sister suspected otherwise.

Mom began to be paranoid, imagining her neighbors breaking into her homoe and stealing old clothes from the basement. At first, we wanted to believe her; we knew that sometimes older people's credibility is questioned because of their age. We wanted to give her the respect that she was due. But finally, when she insisted that a neighbor had climbed through the window to steal the electric bill that she couldn't find, we had the doctor assess her condition. She confirmed that Mom was in the early stages of Alzheimer's.

Should we tell her or not? I came up with the idea of asking her if she wanted to be told. One Sunday, during my usual phone call to her, I asked, "Mom, I was just wondering if, God forbid, you should have cancer or Alzheimer's, or something like that, would you want to know?" "Of course I would want to know!" was her clear reply. A month later we had the doctor tell her. She accepted the information, but seemed unable to absorb it.

Soon, we realized it was not safe for her to stay at home alone. But she would not move; she was adamant. "Charlie is here with me," she would say, our father's name bringing tears to our eyes. Both my sister and I had too much respect for her wishes to move her against her will, but she needed help if she was going to stay. I had to fight with her Medicare HMO to allow for a social work assessment: first, I argued that Alzheimer's was, in fact, a medical condition. Then I argued cost efficiency: it would be more expensive if she injured herself and needed to be hospitalized. Finally, they relented.

The social worker sent to assess my mother was a true professional. He addressed his questions to her rather than to us. My mother was resistant to having anyone in the house, even a home care worker for a few hours each day. He said to her, "I know you want to be independent. Sometimes the way to stay as independent as possible is to get the help you need." She liked and trusted him and agreed to have a worker come in five days a week to help prepare meals and oversee her medications. His approach showed consummate skill—showing her respect, treating her with dignity, acknowledging her overwhelming need for autonomy and independence.

But Mom quickly forgot what she had agreed to during the social worker's visit. We hired someone, but Mom kept fighting with her and "firing" her. We kept convincing her to return—by then, Mom would have forgotten she had "fired" her.

The early stages of Alzheimer's are hardest, I believe, on the person suffering from it. The later stages are hardest on the family. As my daughter said later, "It used to be that she'd be OK and then a fog would come down over her. Now, it seems like the fog is there all the time, and sometimes, for just a brief time, it lifts and she seems like Grandma."

After it became apparent that the part-time worker would not work out, we tried putting Mom into an Alzheimer's unit at a well-respected nursing home. However, at that time she was still physically mobile. The unit really did not meet her needs. Most of the residents were in the later stages of the disease and sat fixed in wheelchairs. Mom was enraged. "Get me out of here! These people are crazy! If you don't take me out, I'll leave and walk home." After three days we got her out, and by some miracle we found a kind woman to live with her. This woman was from Tonga, where the elderly are respected. Over the next three years she, her sister, and then a niece cared for Mom at home until she died. Fortunately my parents had saved money over the years, and we gradually cashed in their CDs to pay for Mom's care.

My sister lived nearby and was able to check on Mom daily and arrange for doctors' appointments, purchase medications, and deal with emergencies. Mom was on several medications, for both congestive heart failure and Alzheimer's. She was losing weight and complained of insomnia. Finally, her doctor determined that the medications were no longer helping her and took her off most, even replacing Coumedin, a blood thinner, with aspirin. Amazingly, she slept better and her appetite returned. "Where is my breakfast?" she'd demand of her helper, not remembering that she had eaten breakfast an hour ago. That wonderful woman wouldn't argue with her, but would simply prepare another breakfast.

My sister and I were able to agree on most details about Mom's care, although I must admit that the roles of older and younger sister sometimes got in the way. It is not unusual that during a parent's last years siblings will replay their childhood relationships. I finally became aware that this was happening between us and was able to recognize my "kid" sister as the able, competent adult she now was.

Several hospitalizations over time caused Mom terrible anxiety and she seemed to mentally deteriorate after each one. She was now entering the last stage of Alzheimer's. She no longer recognized us. She had become physically frail, somewhat incontinent, and almost blind. I knew that most frail elderly who get pneumonia and survive it last, on average, only another six months. My sister and I both agreed that if Mom got pneumonia, we would not send her to a hospital. When, at 89, she contracted pneumonia and we told the doctor our wishes, she arranged for hospice care. Mom died four days later, in her own home, surrounded by her family. It was a good death.

So, what have I learned? Even as a professional, my emotions as a daughter often got in the way of my "professionalism." At a time like this, being a daughter, son, or spouse is one's primary role. It's important to recognize this and to get all the help that is available. It is imperative to continue to treat the person with Alzheimer's with respect and to recognize that she is grasping to maintain control of her own life. Don't argue and try to rationally convince that person. At this point, she is not rational. Like small children, sometimes distractions work better.

It helps to maintain a sense of humor. As they say, sometimes you have to laugh to keep from crying. It's also important to keep your sentences simple—complex sentences confuse them. Don't say, "Do you want to go for a walk or do you want to go shopping?" Just ask, "Do you want to go for a walk?" Work to overcome old patterns of dysfunctional behavior among siblings. Let go of whatever old rivalries and grudges that may lie under the surface of these relationships. Working together on behalf of a loved one is paramount.

Finally, what we realized when Mom was in the late stages and couldn't recognize us is that she would respond to human warmth and to touch. She'd say, "I don't know who you are, but I like you." Her rational processes had shut down, but she could still sense the feeling of love and caring. Although the mother I had known gradually disappeared, I still loved the woman she had become. She may not have known my name, but I know she still loved me.

Ruth is a professor and former Dean of Stony Brook University School of Social Welfare, and is Director of the school's Social Justice Center.

Whoosh!

Judy Kronenfeld

I am on my way to take Dad to the urologist. He has prostate cancer, which he has, of course, forgotten. It is a hot June morning in Southern California after days of marine fog. The jacaranda trees are scattering purple petals like wedding guests showering rice on brides and grooms.

When I get to the assisted living residence, he is not sitting in the chair where someone usually deposits him, this after I've called several times to remind them to remind him to be ready, which, of course, he forgets as soon as he is reminded. I check the other building, where he sometimes goes on his better days in search of some "action": Bingo, the occasional entertainer. Nope. A staff person emerges. Oops, he must have gotten on the bus taking residents to the drugstore. The executive director of the facility radios the bus driver. I drive back to the drugstore (where I have just been, to buy the denture tablets Dad forgets to use) and find him sitting in the facility van. The bus driver hands him over to me.

"We have a doctor's appointment," I say. "Whoosh," he says, his now most characteristic sound—a quick expulsion of breath through loose, slightly inverted lips, a kind of strong sigh. "I didn't know."

He is not entirely steady on his feet, as if he's forgotten for a second what walking is, or maybe he's forgotten where he is, this little shopping center a half-mile from where he lives now. He's wearing the same light-colored jeans—pee stained around the fly—that he was wearing a few days ago when my husband and I took him to dinner, and a few days before that, when I dropped by to give him a new darker blue pair I'd bought.

"Whoosh," he says, getting into the car awkwardly, feet all a-fumble.

"We're going to the doctor," I say.

"Oh. Any particular reason?" he asks.

I explain, roughly, about the prostate cancer.

"Oh, I didn't know," he says.

I turn off the radio that comes on as soon as the car starts. I tell him the upside: he'll just get a manual exam and a hormone shot to control the prostate problem. I don't discuss the radiation treatment possibly looming on the horizon, every day for eight weeks. When the radiation oncologist found out my father was 87, he told me no need for *that*, clearly doing a quick statistical computation. Chances of dying before the cancer kills him? Something or other percent. On the other hand the urologist, who actually looked into my dad's face during three appointments and who knows he's otherwise healthy, suggested that the optimal treatment is hormone therapy *and* radiation, though last time, he did say hormone therapy alone was a "good choice we have made together." I tried to decipher what that was code for.

Now, as we whiz down the boulevard under the blithe opulence of the jacarandas, I try to engage my father's long term memory. I take his left hand in my right; his signature strong squeeze isn't quite forthcoming. What I want to know is how exactly he left Germany in 1934. I know his eldest brother Ben, now long dead, who stowed away on a ship and wound up in the U.S., was the one who arranged visas for my grandparents and my aunt and uncles, now mostly gone or ancient and sick. But it occurred to me that I don't know what the difficulties for a Jew, even a Jew with a visa, leaving the year after Hitler came to power, might have been. But I wind up feeding him more information than he gives me.

"I think I flew," he says.

"In 1934?"

"It must have been a ship, then," my father says. "Ben would know. Whoosh."

We stop for a long light; I have to take my hand back.

"And how is Duvid," my father asks, maybe for the fifth time since I took him off the senior van, sweetening my husband's name, as he always does.

"David's OK," I say.

"And how are the children," he says, also for the fourth or fifth time. I can feel his brain grinding through its gears. "How is Danny," he asks. For a second I imagine my father imagining the children, now flung world-wide, in their beds, still at home.

"He's fine. He's still in Latvia doing research for his Ph.D. in Riga, at least some of the time."

"Oh, that's right," Dad says, "he's in Latvia." The words come off his lips with the aural equivalent of a vacant stare. The gears grind again, this time more protractedly. "And how is Mara," he asks. "She's fine, right"?

"She's still in Morocco," I say.

"That's right. She's in Morocco." My daughter had called this morning. She's packing for her return to the U.S., anxious about the job hunt to come.

"But, they're both happy," he says. "I mean, they're *happy*."

"They're OK," I say.

"Whoosh," my father says. And then, as we enter the parking lot of the medical building, "Oh, we're going to the doctor."

"Yes."

"Any particular reason?" my father asks.

Dad opens the door and shows me into the urologist's office, like a well mannered suitor on a date. There is no one in the waiting room. At first I am afraid they have scheduled him with the male nurse alone while the doctor is in surgery, which would be a problem since I really need the doctor to do that digital exam, to tell me that we can continue to make that "good choice" of hormone therapy "together," at least for now.

I am thinking, selfishly, of how much I want to get away for a couple of weeks this summer, and of how that will be impossible if David—even sweetened David—and I have to alternate taking Dad to radiation therapy every single weekday. Treatment which, despite assurances about how well it is tolerated (by the doctor, who hasn't experienced it), sounds nasty.

Partly in recompense for my thoughts, I reach across to give my Dad's thick, liver-spotted hand a squeeze. I stroke the left side of his bald head, his coarse fringe of white hair. I smile at him. He smiles back with a good-natured, self-effacing grin, as if we have just shared a mild joke at his expense. Reflexive immigrant ingratiation, even with his American-born daughter? Or the intrinsic sweetness of his nature? I still don't know. I give him one of the magazines I have brought along. He studies the cover carefully. Then he scrutinizes an ad on the flip side.

"And how are the children?" he asks.

I repeat what I've already said, adding a bowdlerized version of Mara's job anxieties. What the hell. "She's always had a good head on her shoulders," my father says. "She knows what to do.

Right?" He still sees everything through the permanent rose-colored glasses of his immigrant generation.

Is this cheerful conversation really that different from all my conversations with my father, convinced that his American child and grandchildren possess all the ingredients for success and personal happiness? Now I'm not sure I remember if he's always been like this. How long will my own memories last before they go whoosh? Oh, but I do remember *this*: the optimism, his twenty one gun "smile and the world smiles with you" treatment, applied intensively, hands on, when either grandchild felt low. Odd thing is, it was pretty effective.

I wish my father could smile my son into calling him more often, even if their conversation dims more than it brightens, like a lamp with a bad connection.

Four years from now, on Valentine's day, my son will have a "pure Grandpa moment": he will impulsively duck into a supermarket and buy boxes of chocolate for everyone he works with, the cooks, the drivers, his co-workers, and then go back and get a second box for the drivers, because there are so many of them.

Four years from now an East Coast cousin will call me up and tell me she *must* move closer to her grandchildren. She's just had dinner with my daughter Mara, and she'll say she covets the role Mara's grandfather had in her life. "He was the person with the 'single greatest influence,' your daughter said. I *want* that!"

But now it is June, 2001, and we are waiting in the doctor's examining room, Dad in the one chair, me on an extra stool. "Well, when you write to the children, give them my very best," my father says, putting my magazine down with the pile on the waiting room table. I gently retrieve it.

I have told the male nurse who ushered us in that we hope we can still put off radiation if the doctor thinks the signs are good. He leaves and comes back with Dad's hormone shot, making a joke about schoolgirls sent out into the hall as he sends me out into it. "So, you want to go on radiation," the nurse says confusingly when he opens the door again to let me in. "No," I shake my head. "We want to put it *off*." "I didn't understand a word," Dad says, buckling his belt as the nurse exits. But he seems to sense my exasperation. He gives me that little self-effacing grin as he sits down again in the one chair. He has shaved erratically; there are long hairs under his chin, and some on his upper cheeks. "I feel as if I have one more baby," I say, to him, wiggling his nose with my fingers.

But I want to travel this summer, many summers, while I still can, I am thinking. I want to host gala June weddings for my happy children, when they marry talented, kind, and cute significant others. I want my father, his hair black, to hold the children's hands and mine in his vise-like grip, saying, "See, what did I tell you! They have good heads on their shoulders." I want him to be uncommonly gracious to my long-dead mother as they *kvel* over the grandchildren's *mazel*.

"I hope I don't act like a baby," my father says, turning up the smile wattage. I stroke his bald head. I remember, as a kid, how he let me pull his hair into a fluff on either side of his face; it was our Herr Doktor Einstein game.

At last the doctor arrives. He shakes my father's hand warmly; my father, who has just asked me again what office we are in and who we are seeing, nevertheless looks at him as if he were a long lost *landsman*; a fellow countryman, or the brilliant nephew recommended by a best friend. The doctor immediately launches into a well-meaning but tortured mode of medical speech that is, I think, a measure of his difficulty with being scientifically accurate in language that is understood by ordinary mortals. I glean that my father's blood work is good. I step out again while he does the digital exam.

When I come back, the doctor and I talk about fingers and how accurate they are, while my father, again buckling his belt, continues to beam beatifically. Reprieve, once again reprieve! From whatever it was that lurked in the future. I mumble about "quality of life . . . difficult decisions." The doctor goes on about the sound choice we have arrived at together, at least for the moment, and how we'll re-evaluate in four months, when we may well encounter a change in condition.

A phone rings in the examining room. "I'm not here," my father says gaily.

In the elevator on the way down, his arm in mine, I mumble about long-term decisions. "I'm not complaining," my father says. "I'm an old man. But I'm not complaining." We step out into the dazzling sun.

"I mean as long as you're helping me...."

"No point in talking now then," I say, pressing his arm a little tighter against me, as we negotiate the steps.

"Exactly," he says, righting himself from a slight falter as he transitions to flat ground. Together our eyes scour the parking lot; I spot the car that used to be his and we set off towards it.

"And how are the children?" my father says.

Whoosh.

Judy Kronenfeld's poems have appeared in *Poetry International, The Women's Review of Books, The Portland Review, Spoon River Poetry Review* and in anthologies such as *Red, White & Blues: Poets on the Promise of America*. In addition to her poetry, she has published stories, essays, and a book of scholarship entitled *King Lear and the Naked Truth* (Duke University Press, 1998). She teaches in the Creative Writing Department at the University of California at Riverside.

Alzheimer's, Artichokes, and Forgiveness

Ihla Nation

Alzheimer's Disease is an octopus. Its tentacles stretch out through the ether, strangling the lives of those within its reach. The aftermath of dementia leaves survivors weaving the frayed threads of their lives into lessons colored in grief, anger, fear, sadness, and human frailty.

For me, forgiveness was the most difficult lesson I learned from my mother's Alzheimer's Disease. I easily forgave my mother, whose illness spread slowly like ivy up a wall, hiding her from us. More difficult was forgiveness for my father, who deserted his wife of 35 years when she most needed him, but eventually, I escaped the grasp of anger. I had no need to forgive my brother and sister whose pain was as great as mine, though my brother could no longer visit because "that woman is not my mother." Even God received exoneration for letting Alzheimer's steal my mother's soul long before it stole her body, orphaning me emotionally and spiritually.

It was forgiving myself that became a troublesome, labyrinthine journey. "Forgiveness for what?" my friends asked. I was too ashamed to admit the truth. So I kept it secret, that feeling sorry for myself suffocated compassion for my mother when she confused me with my sister or thought I was a complete stranger; that I was impatient with the endless questions, the constant neediness, the inability to remember how she made those wonderful cinnamon rolls; that I was angry over tradition lost before I had a chance to value it or even realize that it was my mother, now unable to guide me, who carried half of my psychic inheritance. The tears I shed at the end of each visit came from self-pity, not empathy.

Forgiveness is like eating an artichoke. You pluck off a leaf at a time, sometimes slowly, sometimes quickly, but eventually you get to the heart of it. My mother, in the midst of the illness that took her into the Twilight Zone of unrecognizable objects, people, and places, taught me to pull off the first leaf.

The nursing home where she lived frequently moved her around. She often lived in a room only two weeks before she was relocated: her incessant chatter drove roommates to complain. It *was* annoying, but in retrospect I believe she was trying to articulate all the things she needed to say—things her quick-tempered Irish father had not allowed her to say as a child or that women who came of age in the '40s and '50s were expected to keep to themselves. Was she rushing to say all those repressed words before the language center of her brain came unplugged and she never spoke again?

But the continual prattle was irritating, like people talking behind you in a movie. One day Mom's chatter so annoyed a man playing cards in the dining room that he picked up a heavy metal ashtray and threw it at her. It missed and my mother laughed, her lifelong hot nature cooled by mental deterioration. When the nurse's aide informed me, my Irish temper that lay just below the surface raged loose. I turned to stomp self-righteously down the hall to the administrator's office. My mother stopped me.

"It was my fault," she said. "He did tell me to shut up several times."

"That doesn't make it okay, Mom."

"Forget it. He is all alone in the world. He's lost his wife and family, and no one ever comes to visit." Playing cards was one of the only pleasures he had left. Even in the midst of dementia, she understood he was throwing the ashtray not at her, but at the injustice that steered his life so cruelly. Her compassion for his sadness allowed her to forgive his behavior.

It was in that moment, and in all the moments when she did not criticize or condemn us for moving her to a nursing home, for not taking her home when she wanted to go, for my father and brother not visiting her, that the seeds of compassion were planted in me. Though most days she couldn't remember my name, she taught me well. The first leaf pulled from the artichoke of forgiveness eventually led me to the heart of my own absolution.

Forgiveness came in layers. Sometimes it hit a dead-end and I had to accept this might be as much mercy as I had in me. Or I thought forgiving myself or others was a job well done, then a memory would pop like a flashbulb, bringing with it fresh feelings of anger or disappointment. The pain would rise again, and I would need to renew the process of granting pardon.

But each time I thought I was lost in the maze, I discovered I'd only made a wrong turn, I was not back at the beginning. Getting back on track was easier because my compassion for and acceptance of human frailty—even my own—grew with each derailment. With patience, forgiveness grew wide enough and deep enough to include me. The heart of the artichoke was there to savor.

Ihla Nation is a freelance writer who lives in Lafayette, Colorado. Her essays, articles, commentaries and reviews have been published in magazines, newspapers, and online. She has a bachelor's degree in social work from Colorado State University and a masters degree in religious studies from the University of Colorado.

Losing My Father

Brenda van Dyck

"We are the sum of our memories. Everything we know, everything we perceive, every movement we make is shaped by them."

—*David Shenk*, The Forgetting

My dad has Alzheimer's Disease. I've finally gotten used to saying it. In the beginning, it was easier to say that my dad couldn't remember things very well, or that he got easily confused—that happens to a lot of older people. Finally admitting my dad had Alzheimer's Disease was admitting all the things it will eventually do to him. The disease has already taken so much of him away: it's like looking at a jigsaw puzzle; you can make out the whole picture with just a few pieces missing, but when more and more pieces get lost, it's hard to tell what the picture is.

He is no longer the man he was when I was growing up. He no longer fixes things or gardens or cooks or reads. Alzheimer's started taking him away, slowly, years ago. First, he seemed to have a hard time finding words. We would be talking and he would pause, searching, his face turned downward in concentration, his brow furrowed. He would look up and say with slight exasperation, "Ah, I can't think of the word." I would come up with the missing word, interject it for him, and then we could move on with our conversation. Now it is difficult to have any kind of conversation with him. All of his words get stuck, somewhere in his synapses. This is expressive aphasia, and it happens to most people who have Alzheimer's.

At the same time he was losing his words, he began to get confused doing routine things. Once, he went on an errand to the grocery store and asked an employee to help him find an item advertised in the newspaper. When he showed her the ad, she quipped that she would have a hard time showing him where the item was because he was in the wrong store. We—my mother and my siblings—nervously laughed as he told us about it, but to us it was one more piece of evidence that something was wrong.

Sometimes he would say things that wouldn't make any sense. The day after my parents returned from a European vacation, he told me they had been touring the national parks out West. When I tried to tell him where he'd been, he wouldn't believe me. I talked with my mom immediately after that conversation, hoping she would say something that would explain it, that she would give me reassurance that he was okay. She said only, "That just happens sometimes."

Sadly, my father is losing a lifetime of memories truly worth remembering. His early life was marked by poverty and war. He was born to German parents in a Yugoslavian village. Up until a few years ago, he would still tell me with wonder in his voice how happy he was then to get an orange at Christmastime. Just one meager orange, dropped into the bottom of his stocking was enough to delight him. While my father was still young, his father left for Yugoslavia to work in Munich. When he was 12, my father joined him in Munich to learn a trade. At the end of World War II the family who remained in Yugoslavia was evacuated when the German soldiers could no longer protect them. In 1952, at the age of 25, my father immigrated to this country. By the time I was born, the last of his four children, he had been in this country for 15 years. It's these early memories that he most readily recalls as he loses more and more of his mental abilities; they seem to make the most sense to him.

The stories of my father's foreign childhood, his family's poverty, his leaving home to work and his coming to America to make a better life for himself: these are the memories that have shaped *my* life, as well. Having an immigrant father seemed so exotic to me when I was a child. He spoke in a different language and had an accent; he had brothers who lived in Germany. I reveled in the stories he would tell me of growing up in Yugoslavia and Germany.

The reason my father can't remember things is physical. It isn't that he's not trying; effort has nothing to do with it. I wish it were. I think he would do whatever he could to stave off this disease. His German stubbornness would see him through to lucidity, I'm sure of it. That stubbornness has helped him all his life. When he was 14, working as a baker's apprentice in World War II Munich, air raids came almost every night. When the sirens sounded my father would carry his quadriplegic neighbor down four flights of stairs to the bomb shelter of their building. Then he would carry him back up. An hour later, the sirens might go off again, and he would repeat the act. That determination helped him when he started his life over in America. After working so hard to build a happy life here, it isn't right that a disease would take that life away from him.

As my father loses his memory, I turn to memories to think about him. Through a lifetime of memories I see him for who he is and who he once was. He's changed so much his true identity seems to be the most accurate in my memories. He was so capable. It seemed he could do anything. He used to harvest a bevy of vegetables from his garden all summer long, change the oil in the car, bake hearty wheat bread, build things around the house. I miss that man. So many puzzle pieces are gone now that the picture looks entirely different. I can hardly stand to think about it.

The sadness creeps up on me and catches me off guard. Early on in his disease, I attended a class about memory loss sponsored by the Alzheimer's Association. There was a tall, thin old man in front of me, hunched over his cup of weak coffee, flanked by his wife and daughter. I knew instantly that this debilitated man wasn't the man he used to be. It hit me that this is how people see my dad, not for the man he was, but the weak, empty man that Alzheimer's has turned him into. I put my things down and walked to the bathroom crying, thinking I didn't want to be a part of this club. There is little hope in this disease, only ways to cope.

Understanding the science behind Alzheimer's Disease has helped me cope. When comparing the brain of an Alzheimer's patient with a normal brain, the difference is stark. The Alzheimer's brain is noticeably smaller. It is brown and shriveled. As brain cells die, the spaces between the coils of the brain leave wide gaps that shouldn't be there. It's into those spaces that the lost memories and abilities disappear. The disease currently affects about four and a half million Americans. Of people over the age of 65, one in ten has it. It is the seventh leading cause of death in adults, after heart disease, cancer, and stroke. It affects men and women from all socioeconomic parts of society. No one is immune. With no cure or effective prevention, between 11.3 and 16 million Americans are projected to have the disease by 2050. The cause of Alzheimer's is unknown.

The facts bring me face-to-face with the realities of this disease. In the beginning, it was stunning to read through the top ten warning signs of Alzheimer's Disease and see how they fit my dad. "Difficulty performing familiar tasks." Yep. "Problems with language." Yep. "Disorientation as to time and place." Again, yes. "Changes in mood or behavior." Yes. "Loss of initiative." Positive, all positive through the rest of the list. I couldn't deny it was happening. I want to know as much as I can about the disease, but the more I know, the sadder I get. It's part of accepting what is happening, but it also sets me further on the path of grief.

They call Alzheimer's the long goodbye. It's a long, slow process of grieving, as the losses mount up. But it's sneaky—often you don't realize something is missing until it's gone. All of a sudden, it seemed my father didn't know how to use a knife to cut his food or couldn't tie his shoes. With each new loss, as my father becomes less of the man he once was and more dependent on his wife and children, my grief deepens.

It seems especially cruel that a disease would rob a person of memory, because memories are vital for living. They are the key to understanding where we have come from and how we've lived. They provide meaning to the ordinary events of our lives. They work unconsciously to tell us how to function day to day. Memories pop in and out of our minds all day long, their relevance not always apparent. They define us and give context to our lives.

How does memory define us? Memory doesn't shape us, the events of our lives do, but without memory, you can't make sense of your life and the events you've lived through. What takes over when memory leaves and random black spots appear in the picture of your life? Do you fill it with guesswork?

I'm learning to appreciate what it means to live in the moment. In a way, my father is always living in the present. The immediate past has no meaning for him; the future can't be conceived. Only the here and now. There can be something freeing about living this way. Perhaps it means you are free from the past with its pains and struggles, free from worry. That is an optimistic view, of course, because if given the choice, I'm sure my father would prefer to have a full grasp of the past, present, and future.

My father was stern and often crabby when I was growing up, concerned with providing for his family and getting through daily life. The disease has turned him into a sweet old man. When I go home to spend some time with him, he says with enthusiasm, "Well, thanks for coming over!" And he means it. He's been kissing me on the cheek when I greet him; he never did that before.

His hugs have become hardier, too. We have a litany of goodbyes: "Aufweidersehen," one says. Then the other, "Weidersehen mach fruede," which roughly translates into something like, "Take care until I see you again."

I'm not ready to let him go just yet. As he slips away, I will know who he once was. And I will remember.

———————

Brenda is a writer and editor living in Minneapolis, Minnesota. She is inspired by the words of German artist Käthe Kollwitz: "I am groping in my art, and who knows, I may find what I seek." Brenda has a Master's Degree in Fine Arts with a creative nonfiction writing emphasis from Hamline University in St. Paul, Minnesota.

Dad's Private Police

Catherine A. Johnson

Just over a year ago, my father began telling strange tales of being kidnapped and secretly videotaped. He talked much like my mother did in the later stages of her struggle with Alzheimer's Disease. I was sure we were heading down the same path. The staff at his care facility noted the behavior and lived with it; they could do nothing for him. It was only when he was admitted to the hospital with chest pain that I was able to help bring my Dad some peace and comfort.

He suffered a mild heart attack and was taken by the staff to the hospital. I received the call at 7:30 a.m. that morning and headed to the emergency room. Removing an 87 year-old man from his familiar surroundings, routines and medications is a dicey matter, to say the least. The hours it took for admission did not help matters. While we waited, my father told me that a man, sitting outside the window of the examination room, was cleansing his blood through a tube in his arm. The man he was referring to was working at a computer screen. My father was amazed and thrilled with this new blood cleaning technology.

When he was finally taken upstairs to coronary care, I went outside to call my siblings. Upon my return, everything had changed. He was no longer passive and cooperative. The unfamiliar room had become a dangerous place to him. I found him sitting on the edge of the bed, pale and wide-eyed, taking swings at the nurses to keep them back.

"Oh, Cath!" he cried. "That man over there (pointing at his roommate), he has drugs and booze and he has people in the hall coming to kill me!" When I tried to calm him, he persisted. "Cath you don't know...you have to call the police, get security!" How it hurt to see him so very terrified. He calmed down only when I promised to stay with him and keep watch.

All afternoon I sat and watched him as he lay sedated and huddled under his blanket. My hero, the strongest man in my life, was a terrified little boy who whispered while pointing at people who weren't there. It broke my heart. My presence was not enough to calm him and neither were sedatives.

The stories he told persisted, each one more wild and frantic than the previous. Upon my return from getting something to eat, he was pointing out the door at a man in the hall who was sneaking up to kill him. He said there were people outside the third floor window with machine guns; he urged me to duck. I wanted to ease his fears but it was apparent that even my staying with him all night was not going to do it. The nurses decided to move him to a single room near their station, in the hope of giving him some relief. That is when I saw a possible band-aid for his notions of being the target of gangsters.

My town is home to a very large prison and this hospital cares for its inmates. In the next room was an inmate being watched by two prison guards, both in uniform, packing weapons and badges. Could I? Would they? What the heck. I called to the two rather large young men and the smaller one came to the door.

"Listen, my 87 year old father is being moved to this room because he is sure someone is out to kill him," I explained. "If I told him you were here to protect him as his personal bodyguards would you go along?"

The officer grinned. "Sure, be glad to."

So when they wheeled my father's bed down the hall, I had them stop the bed just outside the door and said, "Dad, you asked me to call the police, now I want you to see." I waved the officers over. They stood on each side of his bed, one bigger than the other, hands on guns, badges shining. "Dad, these officers are here to protect you. They are your own personal police and will be here all night."

"Yes, sir that's right," said one as he tapped Dad's knee.

My Dad's eyes welled with tears as he looked over at me. "Good boys.... Good boys." he said in a cracking voice. I thanked the officers as my father was wheeled into his new room. I doubted whether this helped Dad sleep—I am sure he was still watching the windows—but he did know he had someone to call who had guns at the ready to protect him. And for me, well, the important thing was that I'd done something, and when you watch a loved one suffering, you just want to do...something.

While she and her husband of 32 years were raising three teenage children, Catherine also helped care for her mother, who died from Alzheimer's in 2000. Since her mother's death, writing has helped her to express her emotions and preserve precious family memories. She has published other short stories and essays on family life. She lives in Michigan.

The Art of Memory and Belonging

Tovli Simiryan

We were planning Mama's citizenship day. She had arrived with her son and husband as refugees from the Soviet Union eight years earlier. This day she was scheduled to visit the immigration and naturalization office in Buffalo, New York. She was nervous. That year her memory began to betray her and she was sure the United States would find her unworthy of citizenship and deport her.

The examiner was a kind man. He called our name and we pushed Mama's wheel chair into his tiny office. Rumors had circulated within the Russian community that elders who'd accompanied their children as refugees would no longer have the English language requirements of citizenship automatically waived; if they could not pass the verbal test in English they could be deported.

Mama tried to learn English her first two years in America. She would learn a few words, but small strokes would erase her memory and she would start again. We practiced short sentences, followed by history lessons. Her favorite was *Martin Luther King Jr.*

"What a strong, good face he has," she would say, "his eyes and spirit are clean. Where does he live?" When the sad story of Martin Luther King Jr. was told to her, Mama cried and lamented,

"Even in America, freedom has a price." She was sure Lincoln was Jewish. "Look at his face; that face is Jewish and why would a non-Jewish mother name a child 'Abraham' unless they were Jewish?"

It was enjoyable studying with Mama. Being an American was a source of pride for her. Belonging and freedom were not to be taken for granted. At first, every Friday morning was scheduled as *test day*:

"Mama. Who is the president of the United States?"

"Beel Cleeenton."

"Who is the Mayor?"

"Beel Johns-tun."

"What is the English word for *Duma*?"

"Conk-kress."

It was precious. She fired off responses while hiding her *HAIS— You Are a Citizen* workbook to prove she knew and remembered the answers.

It was just after the Passover holiday one year when Mama began to become confused, forgetting little phrases of her new language and bits of the history of her new culture. Bill Clinton was mistaken for Avraham Avinu; Abraham Lincoln drew a long, deliberate stare, followed by an outburst of anger.

But on this day, we were at the Citizenship Office and there was no turning back. Mama sat in front of the kind man who sorted through applications, asked for signatures and looked Mama in the eye.

"Your mother does not speak English." It was more of a statement than a question. Mama sat in her wheel chair. Her bony hand gripped the prayer book she had carried since her childhood and she shook her hands toward the ceiling as though begging God for mercy.

"She is in her nineties," the examiner noted. "She is a Holocaust survivor, I see. She survived Stalin and was a nurse for thirty years following World War II. She has seen it all, I'll bet. She must have some real memories and stories." The examiner reached into his side drawer and took out a special tool that pressed an embossed stamp on Mama's citizenship papers. He looked at my husband and smiled.

"We will be waiving the language requirement. Congratulations. Your mother has received approval for citizenship." The kind bureaucrat did not receive the sigh of relief he anticipated and looked at my husband with curiosity.

"Is something wrong?"

"No, we are grateful. But my mother, well, she has worked hard all her life and does not expect to be given something for free. If we leave without your asking a few questions, she will not believe she has been accepted as an American." The examiner looked at Mama. Without hesitation he advised, "Ask her in Russian who the president is."

"Mama," "Kto prezident Amerikee; who is the President of the United States?"

"Beel Cleeenton."

The examiner smiled. "Ask her how many senators the state of New York has."

"Mama, how many senators does New York have?"

"*Dva*", she answered in Russian, then corrected herself. "Oy, two."

Before the examiner could ask another question, Mama exploded with every answer to any question about American history she'd ever learned. She was still reciting the names of states as we pushed her out the door, leaving the smiling examiner to continue his day.

It was one of the last days Mama's memory would be available to her. It was not long after Citizenship Day that the strange, glassy stare of dementia showed from her eyes. One minute the strong, demanding nurse from Bendery, Moldova would be singing her childhood songs in Yiddish. She would laugh and joke. She would plan her garden for spring and decide her daughter-in-law could not wash a floor properly and begin this chore each morning at six a.m., before anyone could stop her. She would tell the story of her nursing days, when she and only she correctly diagnosed an ecotopic pregnancy, saving her patient's life. Then, without warning, she was suddenly sure every vineyard in America had been poisoned and we'd spend our evening frantically removing anything remotely associated with grapes from the entire house.

One morning, it became chocolate bars. A chocolate bar needed to be on her dresser at all times or her heart would stop. There was no reasoning with her. My husband and I bought them by the case and each evening we made sure a chocolate bar was within her grasp. She would eat one small piece and place the remaining chocolate beneath her mattress. It was months before we figured out our mysterious problem with ants.

Chocolate bars soon gave way to eye drops. Mama decided that a special bottle of eye drops that had been given to her by a Russian doctor before her son was born would keep her from going blind. We spent hours begging her to describe the bottle and the more we investigated, the angrier she became. We bought every bottle of eye drops available and none was acceptable. Finally, we were given a used amber bottle from one of the Russian elders and had the pharmacist sterilize it and fill it with saline solution. Mama was overjoyed. But the more ideas we came up with to console her and meet her strange, illogical demands, the more pervasive the memory loss, the forgetfulness and rages became.

At first, we ignored the odd behavior, deciding that this was the way old Moldavian nurses age. The blank stares were excused as exhaustion; anger was simply frustration. It was hard to admit, but the stoic elder—Holocaust survivor, witness to Russia's pogroms, the uncompromising woman who'd fled Moldova for Kazakhstan with Nazis in pursuit, deliverer of special potions to her neighbors during the days of poverty that brought Russia to its knees—was losing the ability to remember who she was and what she stood for. Dementia was stealing Mama from us. It crept into our lives like a nightmare but could not be forgotten with the arrival of a sunny morning. This nurse, trained by the Russian military, who had cared for her entire family and had seen the twentieth century come and go, could no longer distinguish day from night.

"*Dai mne Holodilnik...* give me the refrigerator," she often demanded. And when I stood dumbfounded, trying to figure how I'd get the refrigerator upstairs to please her, she became angry. "*Policia, Policia.* Nurse Ester needs you." Mama would yell into the hallway, then navigate to the window where she would bang on the glass pane, alerting the KGB to arrest her poorly behaved and useless children. It took time to realize it was not the refrigerator she was asking for, but her nice, warm robe. The woman who had survived so much, who was literate in five languages, was betrayed by her brain's inability to make words meaningful and useful. No matter how clever we were at figuring out her needs and demands, the confusion continued until the day came when she had trouble recognizing her beloved son.

Mama's son began to see her blank eyes, the loss of memory, confusion and inconsolable anger. It was loss beyond loss for him. It was saying goodbye to the person who'd taught him who and what he was. The brain of this great woman had been attacked with a pervasive disease that affected not only its victim, but the memories of her loved ones.

Who in your life has loved you unconditionally? Picture this person in your mind's eye, focus on their face, the feelings of acceptance, belonging, importance and purpose you experienced. Take a minute and absorb these feelings, magnify them. Then say to yourself, once your heart has filled with this deep, accepting love: *this is who I really am; this is what I am all about.* This is what Mama offered her son and her recently acquired daughter-in-law. She was what life was all about: acceptance, perseverance, compassion, commitment, dignity, balance and history. Now, Mama, the matriarch, was disappearing, day by day, memory by memory and story by story.

"Mama, when is the anniversary of Papa's leaving this world?" her son asked one day. His mother could not remember being married.

"Mama, what was the name of the girl you nursed back to health the winter that was so cold medicine could not be delivered to the rural areas?" Our mother could not recall her life as a nurse.

"Mama, tell us about the Muslim family who hid you from the Nazis and saved your life." Our elderly mother could not recall the months she ran for her life and hid from the Germans in Kazakhstan.

Soon Mama began to fill the loss of memory with made up stories. A "Dr. Rosa" entered our life. Where he came from, my husband and I could never be sure. He appeared because Mama could not recall the name of her American doctor. She decided to call him Dr. Rosa. Soon the character became more complex and appeared whenever her children were slow to meet or understand her needs. Mama would summon Dr. Rosa, who would fire us for incompetence and suggest we consider working in "another hospital". One day, I had disappointed Mama so profoundly that she explained to her son, "Don't even look for your wife, Dr. Rosa has deported her and they have already taken her away."

As the story continued, we discovered Dr. Rosa had two children, Shelomo and Sima, who lived in Mama's two by two foot closet. Soon, Sergei joined the household and anytime our pet dog entered Mama's room, she called for Sergei to shoot the poor animal. Mama hired a chauffeur named Ivan and when she required something from the store we could not provide, she simply called Ivan and he would drive to the store with instructions to say the name, *Ester, the nurse of Bendery* and all of Mama's needs would be met. The characters kept coming and all we could do was enjoy the drama.

Her son, a pragmatic mathematician and computer programmer, needed to make sense of these strange performances. Or maybe it was his attempt to stop the disease and demand that God return his mother to him. At any rate, one evening he had had enough and denied Dr. Rosa's existence, sending Mama into an eloquent fit that resulted in her throwing a variety of cherished possessions against the wall and contacting the KGB to deport us both. He stooped to pick up the pieces of the new telephone Mama had thrown and held them in his hand, showing his ninety-plus year old mother her crime. I guess he'd forgotten Mama had lost her vision and could not see the palm sized electronic corpse.

Rationalism allows us to recognize what has been passed from parent to child; it bestows us with belief in immortality, purpose and continuation. When the keepers of our pasts have forgotten purpose and self, the understanding of what it means to be mortal hits like a war within our souls.

Mama still lives in our home and is approaching her 100th birthday. She continues to visit with Dr. Rosa, she asks for refrigerators instead of warm robes; the KGB has not actually contacted either her son or me and Mama often falls into a strange sleep that seems to last for days.

Occasionally, my husband and I will be downstairs, cooking, cleaning and wondering if Alzheimer's is contagious. Once in a great while, without warning, we hear a strange sound, familiar yet unexpected. We realize it is Mama, singing her childhood songs. Her Yiddish fills every corner of her room and spills into the entire house. We run to her room and see her well mapped face smiling with wisdom, compounded with endurance. If we listen very carefully, if we keep our voices soft and still, she begins to remember her stories. She beckons for Dr. Rosa and her children to come close. My husband and I eavesdrop, and before long we recall our purpose, who we are, where we came from, who we have become and what will become of us.

Tovli "Linnie" Simiryan lives and writes in West Virginia. Her poetry and fiction have appeared in several literary and other publications. A collection of poetry, *The Breaking of the Glass* and a meditation manual, *Ruach of the Elders: Spiritual Teachings of the Silent* will be released in 2007.

Part II

THE SPOUSES

Love is the condition in which the happiness of another person is essential to your own.

—*Robert A. Hemlein*

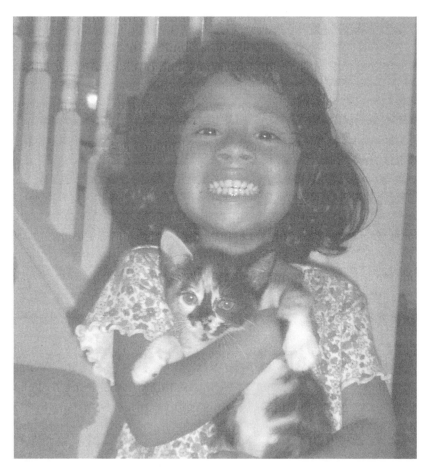

Lucy Shore, page 149

Rebirth

Barbara Pearson Arau

He was once a different person, witty, charming, creative, and smart. Now he is someone else. He has been reborn, and he is not even aware of his metamorphosis.

It started so slowly that I hardly noticed. One day he was speaking normally, the next he was asking me about an old bench he wanted to refinish, a bench we had gotten rid of long ago. When I reminded him of this, he snapped that the bench was in the garage, and why was I being so stupid? My feelings hurt, I left the room. When I returned, he had forgotten all about it. I didn't realized that in the coming weeks and months my feelings would be crushed time and time again, that I would gradually form a shell around them until I became so tough that I could be neither hurt nor touched.

He waits throughout each day, some long, some blessedly short. I look at him now, sitting in his chair by the window in the place that has been his home for the past year, waiting for I know not what. Compassion has returned; he can no longer say mean things to me. In fact, he can no longer say much at all. And so I can forgive the bitter tongue-lashings, the unfounded accusations, the striking out with an open hand. Those were the actions of an unfeeling stranger.

The realization that he was sick took time. I wish now that I had recognized his symptoms in the early stages, that I had asked a doctor about them or understood the signs of oncoming Alzheimer's Disease. What a waste of time it was, his and mine, for me to become resentful and wounded at the injustice of his behavior toward me. Hadn't I always been loving, supportive? What had I done to deserve such cruelty?

I hadn't done anything, of course. As he continued to behave erratically, as others began to notice and comment, I finally woke up and saw him in a new light. My old friend, my best friend, had disappeared. This new person looked the same, had the same voice and the same gestures, but that's where the resemblance ended. The disease progressed inexorably and he regressed, inexorably. He became expert at covering up, compensating for his forgetfulness and loss of recent memory. If I tried to test him, to ask him what year it was or who was president, he would scoff and say everyone knows that. He lost his sense of humor, his curiosity, his ability to read, his wit. Finally, sadly, he completely lost his bearings. I took him to a place where he could be professionally cared for.

He knows me sometimes, I think. He's very polite when he talks. He mostly lives in some faraway, pleasant memory where I've never been, but he seems happy there. Or at least he is calm. I look at him and I try to see him as he once was, but then I realize that's impossible now. He has been reborn into someone else, someone I've never known.

And I think to myself, that's OK. This facsimile person is living a life that belongs only to him and he looks contented. I can deal with this, bringing him cookies and lemonade, trying to make conversation, smiling at his attempts to wave a polite goodbye when I leave, because I know that I can resurrect the original whenever I wish. My memories are sharp and clear, and as long as I have them, he will remain the vibrant, loving, devoted and steadfast man that I married.

During her varied career, Barbara has served as editor of the *Outdoor Life Book Club* and as a copyeditor at New York City and Miami advertising agencies. Her writing has been published in *Bride's*, *Harper's Bazaar*, *Endless Vacation*, *Family Circle*, *The Miami Herald*, *Travel/Holiday*, *International Mystery Journal* and others. Her mystery novel, *Someone's in the Kitchen with Dinah* was published in 2001; she is currently working on a sequel.

Letting Go

Elizabeth Van Ingen

I heard the car screech out and the garage door roll shut. I sank into a chair at the kitchen table and hid my face in my hands. Let him stay at the Holiday Inn. He'd be all right. It was only a mile and a half down the road. What could I do anyway? Frankly, I was glad he was gone. Where is the sweet but sad love story, I thought? This is terror, every day. In the stillness of the kitchen, I reminded myself that I was with him because I chose to be.

My husband was sick. After a long struggle with doctors to have my fears about Tony's symptoms taken seriously, at the age of 67 he was diagnosed with probable Alzheimer's Disease. The disconnect growing between us was not a marital problem that could be fixed, as one doctor suggested, but the result of the disease, which could not be.

The diagnosis did not bring the closure I had expected, but more ambiguity and an overwhelming sense of abandonment. Where were the directions for the rest of my life? I had followed Tony's lead for forty years, literally around the world. Now I had to make the decisions about our future and he wouldn't be able to help me. He didn't respond to me in the loving way he used to. I was fading from his awareness. I stopped expecting any emotional support from him. If I hadn't, every hour of every day would have been a battle.

"I don't know if I can do this, Hanna," I said to Tony's sister. "I am not the nurse type. I can't stand to see Tony so bewildered and angry and out of control. I feel like I'm walking blindfolded, knee deep in mud. I am just stuck."

Her empathy came through the phone as she listened. Then she said, "You don't have to do it, Liz. You can leave; get someone else to take care of him. There are resources. There are homes," and finally, "Some people even divorce."

For a minute, I couldn't speak. "Oh, Hanna," I cried, "He's my husband ... forty years ... I love him. I could never leave him." Was that too quick a decision, I thought as I put down the phone?

When Tony snapped off the TV while I was watching a program, I stifled my reaction and told myself it really wasn't important. Peace was more important to me than a battle over things that didn't matter, and now, nothing mattered. When he shoved a newspaper between my nose and the book I was reading, or demanded my attention while I was on the phone, or adjusted the curtains I had just arranged, I smiled and said nothing. It really didn't matter. When we planned to leave at 9 AM for the two-and-a-half hour drive to Des Moines to our daughter's house for Christmas, it didn't really matter that we left at noon and delayed her plans by three hours. She and I learned to make flexible plans. He hadn't participated in Christmas for years. "What's Christmas anyhow? Christmas is for stupid people. Go by yourself," he said, throwing the keys and kicking the door.

As I let my work and my interests lose their meaning for me, our life slowed to a near standstill. I thought of myself as having been in a speeding car going 75 miles an hour down the highway, then coming to the outskirts of a town and slowing to 45, then 35, then 25. Now, 15 miles an hour felt comfortable and I was old. I was 61 and old and stuck. We were slipping into a troubled new world, he and I, and no amount of money, education, past history, common sense or love could keep us out. I looked to his side of the bed where that morning he had sat, holding his head in his hands whispering, "My brain isn't working; my brain just isn't working. I feel like a balloon floating this way and that with no one holding the string."

My heart wept. He was losing his mind and I ached to gain control. I stood up from the kitchen table, turned out a few lights and got myself into bed. I wore my bathrobe and socks in bed; I was shivering. I lay on my back staring into the dimness, wondering if I should call the Holiday Inn to see if he had gotten there. No, leave him alone, I thought. Quit interfering. He had to rely on me and yet my presence constantly reminded him that he was losing his mind. "No, not in that drawer," I'd say, "The top drawer, the top drawer." "You don't want to eat now; we just ate." "Get ready; we're leaving in five minutes." My constant help must drive him crazy.

I knew his storming out of the house was not my fault, but something I did had triggered it. I tried to control everything, but I had slipped up. My whole body ached as I lay there remembering. Tony had come downstairs to where I was working in my office in our basement. His calendar was in his hand. He stretched out on the couch and said, "Next week we have to get our tickets for Europe to see my mother, make arrangements for our trip to Holland. Are you with me on this?"

"Trip to Europe?" I said, "No, not really. I don't know if we can manage that." He leaped off the couch, fists in the air. "You're always double crossing me! I'll go without you! I can find some lady to go with me! You stay here by yourself! I'm going to do what I want!" He charged at me, red faced, finger pointing, fury and madness spewing out of him. "I can't take it! I can't take you! You're always crossing me! I'll do what I want! I want to see my mother. I'll just get out! I'm leaving!"

He raged up the stairs to the kitchen. I sat for a moment to get my breath and gain control. I closed my work on the computer. Then

I started quietly up the stairs as Tony was at the kitchen door to the garage, slamming around.

"I've already checked in at the Holiday Inn," he yelled, "I'm going."

"Sweetheart..." I started, and he slammed the door behind himself. Gone.

"Sweetheart ...."

What could I have done? I drifted into a fragile sleep, the light still on beside the bed.

A thumping sound came from the front hall and I threw off the covers and ran to open the door. Tony was on his knees, head down, arms up, fists pounding the door so hard that when I opened it he literally rolled in and onto his back, arms and legs flailing uncontrollably.

"I'm going crazy! I don't know where I am! Where am I? I'm going totally crazy! Just kill me! There's no reason to live! You're driving me out of my mind!" His head whipped from side to side. His arms and legs stabbed at the air. Unearthly sounds came from his throat. I backed away, terrified. When he relaxed, I got down on my hands and knees and held him tight, whimpering, half crying, "You're home. It's your home. You're safe. I'm here. I'll never leave you. You're not going crazy. I love you. I love you."

Then fury struck again and I jumped back, afraid of his thrashing limbs. "Just kill me! I'm going crazy!" He grabbed at the railing, which divided the hall from the sunken living room. Then he let go, falling back and whispering, "Just kill me. I'm going crazy." We sat like that crying and screaming for a long, long time. Eventually, Tony struggled to his feet and leaned on me. We shuffled to the bedroom. I took off his clothes and shoes and got him into bed. It was 3:30 in the morning.

"Why did I leave?" he asked, "What made me leave the house?"

"Just relax," I said, "It's over now. You can rest." I didn't want him to remember. But he did.

"You wouldn't let me see my mother!" Like a volcano, his rage came again, spewing out anger and confusion, his arms and legs jabbing like spears of lightning. I stood at a physically safe distance, but I felt burning heat flow over me.

"I'm exhausted," he said abruptly, and slept.

I did not. I threw on jeans and a sweatshirt and huddled at my desk with the phone. I needed help. I was afraid. My mother's words played in my mind, "You can handle it, Liz. I know you can handle it." Tony needed me now more than he ever had. I was his conduit to the world, to help, to comfort, to love. I was not helpless. I was not postponing my life. This was my life, the life I had chosen when I married him, and chosen again when I knew he was sick. I breathed deeply and shifted from a state of fear to a "handling-it" mode. Not waiting for offices to open, I picked up the phone in those early morning hours and left messages with doctors and organizations that could help.

By nine o'clock that morning, I had talked with our neurologist. When I described the incident to him he asked, "Had Tony been drinking?"

"No," I answered. No? He had been at the Holiday Inn bar for five hours. No? What was I thinking? Was I thinking? I had read and been told that Alzheimer's patients should stay away from alcohol, but I thought, what the hell? Life is over anyway, what difference could a glass or two of wine make? Now I knew that alcohol could have a devastating effect when combined with Alzheimer's.

By 9:30, our friend Don, a real estate person, was at the house to give me an appraisal on our property. I knew we couldn't stay here in a big house on an acre of lawn and garden, with no help or family nearby, and with Tony presenting such unpredictable behavior. Don and I stood in the driveway talking. I told him about Tony's illness and the frightening episode of the night before.

At 9:45, Tony came out into the sunshine, dressed, shaved, hair combed, smiling and greeting Don as though nothing had happened. I looked at him from across the driveway. I saw the man I knew so well, straight and tall and handsome. I was overcome with love and compassion for him. No one would guess he had a terrible, mind-destroying disease.

I felt confident enough to plan that trip to Holland where Tony was born and had lived until he was twenty-one. In Amsterdam, in between visits with his mother in the nursing home, we strolled along the canals, holding hands and stopping to eat Dutch pancakes and fried eggs with thin roast beef on fresh white bread. He showed off to me by speaking Dutch, German, and French. At night we held each other tight under a fluffy down comforter.

But it was evident that the dementia was progressing. "Don't tell me. I know. Our room is on the right," he said, as I steered him to our hotel room on the left. "Where are my, you know, my things?" he asked, looking for his underwear to pack in his already packed suitcase. "Oh, ha, ha! That's not where I want to go!" he said, opening the door to the hall, looking for the bathroom. He woke me in the night by sitting straight up in bed and remarking on the flowers climbing up the walls or the bicycle on the bedside table. He, who had traveled the world all of his life, was in a land more foreign than he had ever been, and I was the guide. "Well, you know, the women do everything now-a-days," he excused himself as I ordered his meals, paid the bills and handled the tickets. Sadly, two weeks after our return, he forgot that we had seen his mother.

My level of acceptance of his illness grew, but I never knew how sick he was. He was always a little farther into the disease than my acceptance would allow. I was still looking for a plan of action, or some way to gain control of the chaos and to protect him from his disease. I accepted his behavior as it was at that moment and his life became my life. It was what I wanted to do, but it cost me.

For a few years, medication tempered Tony's rages of frustration, but inevitably his diseased brain deteriorated to the point where he had no control over behavior, no ability to recognize people or objects, and though he talked incessantly, no understanding of language. I found the help we both needed by placing him in an Alzheimer's nursing home. Two months later, when he was in the dining room of the facility, standing tall, greeting people and arranging chairs, a visiting Hospice nurse saw him and recognized signs of approaching death. Tony had developed an infection in a saliva gland which, if not treated, would spread and kill him.

He had shown me he wanted to leave years ago on that night he had slammed out the kitchen door. I knew he wanted to get away and be free of the disease, so this choice was not a difficult one. I allowed Hospice to help him go in peace and comfort.

Ultimately, of course, it was not my choice; his life was not in my control or his. Alzheimer's had taken over long ago. My choice was to provide love, respect, understanding and, lacking a road map, to seek out the best road, to soften the sharp curves and walk beside him as far as I could go.

Elizabeth was born in San Francisco and graduated from the University of California at Berkeley. She met her husband, a native of Holland, in Teheran in 1959, where she was teaching fifth grade at the American School. She now lives in the Denver area.

Before His Time: The Strange Case of the Missing Salmon

Maggie B. Dickinson

In 1996 we set off from Kalamata airport in a hired car and spent three glorious days exploring the southern Peloponnesus of the Greek mainland. I'd dreamed of this journey for years. It was well worth every second of that wait, and I was blissful as we headed north via the rugged western edge of the Mani peninsula to a resort called Stoupa. The sun was hitting the ocean as we cruised into the golden bay that would be our base for the remainder of the holiday. And then, in a single sentence, he killed the holiday mood. The words Jim used confirmed what I had been refusing to face for a long time: "I can't remember the name of a single place we've visited," he confessed. And so began the battle with Alzheimer's Disease.

Within a few months of arriving back home in England he'd lost his job, which was hardly surprising, since he had a managerial position and his deteriorating memory had been giving rise to increasing concern.

Navigation problems came next. We'd arrive at a road junction in an area he knew well, and he'd say, "Which way?" The first time it happened I laughed and told him to stop joking, but when I turned and looked at his profile I could see his jaw was set. What must it have been like for him to feel lost, to be heading into an uncertain and confusing world but be incapable of articulating his fears to his nearest and dearest because of a growing inability to express himself?

We'd both started employment at the age of 15 in a culture that subscribed to a strong work ethic. We were brought up to carry on despite illnesses; to recuperate on weekends. Retirement was the carrot. All our lives we chased it with the promise of pensions and time to enjoy the fruits of our labors. I had a whole shelf full of books on Europe in readiness. Maybe we'd buy a camper van. Perhaps we'd take a backpack of casual clothing and go island-hopping in Greece, or fly to the French Riviera and use the fast TGV trains at will.

I can recall the sheer bitterness I felt about our situation in general, and towards Jim in particular. Not only had a lifetime of dreams been shattered but the retirement for which I'd always yearned had been cancelled. As if the blow of his illness were not enough, the loss of his income was a further burden. For almost a year, while it was still safe to leave him unsupervised, Jim stayed at home as I continued to work. But despite my pleadings, he steadfastly refused to see a consultant and clung to our family doctor's theory that he could be suffering from stress.

Unknown to Jim, I eventually confronted his doctor and suggested we trick him into a consultation. When we finally saw a neurologist, the diagnosis came as no surprise, but I was grateful that Jim was immediately prescribed the cognitive enhancer Aricept, which greatly slowed the progress of his illness.

A person under the age of 65 who is diagnosed with Alzheimer's is classified as having early-onset dementia. Sadly, there are instances of Alzheimer's Disease among those who have small children or still have young people to put through college. Consequently, early-onset Alzheimer's, while having plenty in common with other dementias in the way it presents itself, brings a different set of problems because of the younger age and consequent needs of its victims.

At that time, there was scant consideration of the quality of the life of early-onset victims and little available day care. I was particularly concerned about Jim's ego and dignity, both of which had taken a nosedive. Despite a desperate need to recover my own personal space that he'd invaded—it felt as if he were grafted to my hip—I would not send him to the usual form of day care, where everyone was ten to twenty years his senior. He was already depressed enough by his situation without adding further insult.

In time, I discovered a hospital where a Reminiscence Therapy day care program operated, and it proved to be our lifeline, for he loved it, especially as there were several people his own age with whom he could identify, as well as a very caring staff to whom he could tell his worries. Instead of merely being a "minding" service, there was a structured program and a decent range of activities, such as dancing, listening to music from our youth, trips to farms and other interesting venues. He came home thoroughly stimulated and content, not least because he'd been able to show other members of the group how to play pool. He'd been in a safe environment that held no threats, which boosted his confidence.

Jim grew younger. His favorite companion became our granddaughter, aged two. One day as I supervised them, I realized that I had lost him forever, that he was never coming back. Not only had he become my child, I had reluctantly taken on the role of mother. The real problem here was not that I couldn't chastise him for being naughty or stand him in the corner but that I suspected he was going to get a lot more difficult to handle.

Nobody asked me if I wanted to be his caregiver, and I resented that, as I resented him wearing three shirts simultaneously or changing clothes several times a day. I wanted to be his wife, his lover, his best friend—like before. Instead, we were treading a rocky and precipitous path to an unknown and daunting destination. Every day presented us with new challenges, and I dealt with them in whatever way my capabilities allowed.

It takes a great deal of patience to cope with whatever problems arise from dementia; take, for example, The Case of the Missing Salmon. I was poaching a large fillet on the stove and had left the chore for less than a minute to go upstairs for a towel. When I returned, Jim was washing out the pan. "Salmon? What salmon? I don't know what you're talking about," he said. I never found the fish: he must have opened the door and thrown it over the garden fence. It might keep company somewhere with a four pack of beer, a bottle of ketchup, and a host of other groceries that disappeared into thin air.

There was an endless list of missing objects, some eventually found as part of his hidden treasure troves, like my mobile telephone and spectacles, and some never to surface again, such as the TV remote control, nail scissors, tweezers, a new lipstick and several door keys. They fall within the "magpie" or "squirrel" syndrome that affects dementia sufferers and prompts them to hide items, the act probably triggered by an instinct to put something away for a rainy day. Frequently it didn't make sense, like the shriveled black banana skins, four tarnished horse brasses, and a pile of currency that I discovered on a high shelf in the kitchen when I was cleaning in readiness for moving out of the cottage.

I learned a valuable lesson from that salmon incident. Instead of reprimanding him, which would have been a waste of time and upsetting to us both, I shrugged my shoulders, said *qué será será*, and rustled up poached eggs on toast instead. Preserving a sense of humor was one of my biggest challenges in the early days, but in time it came back to the fore where it's always been, and I began to see the comical aspect of many scenarios. A typical example was the day, quite soon into the illness, when I didn't realize how far his confusion and memory loss had progressed. I'd bought him a tin of paint to spruce up the front of the cottage. He just loved to paint. I got sidetracked with household jobs and forgot to check on him. Less than an hour later a neighbor flew in to say that he wasn't doing our property at all but *the cottage next door* instead, and his handiwork was all too obvious! I didn't laugh at the time, but it's a tale that has lightened many a conversation in recent years. I don't feel in the least as though I've betrayed Jim when I tell the story; he'd have laughed a lot louder than anyone else, for laughing was a skill at which we both excelled.

Fortunately, a daunting period when he became suspicious and distrustful was short lived. Then, every morning there was a race to the letter box, because he wanted to open all the mail. He became almost paranoid about money, too, which was totally out of character. Each time we went into town, he wanted to draw cash out of the bank's dispenser with his card. This fixation with cash, and his accurate recall of his pin number, became quite scary, because the money invariably went missing even though he was rarely out of my sight. Fortunately he could only draw amounts that I supervised, for I couldn't let him have sole charge of the transaction or we might have been left without any funds at all. I later discovered he'd hidden the money with those banana skins. This, like many more issues, was not without solution, for I threw his card on the stove when he wasn't looking, and he forgot all about it within a matter of days.

Caregivers involved with dementia need to ensure that their own mental health remains intact and that they get relief not only through day care, but respite care, too, so that there is an opportunity for breaks that last a few days or even a week, especially away from home. As the various care programs gave me some time for myself, I managed to pursue a few hobbies on a small scale and had the occasional opportunity to visit or dine out with friends. I even had several weekend breaks that were arranged especially for caregivers. The change of environment, a program of interesting events, and the company of others who were in a similar position allowed me to thoroughly recharged my batteries.

A turning point came on the 13th of October, 1999. I'd foolishly booked a holiday for the two of us on the Greek island of Crete. We never got there, because the pains I experienced in my left arm that day while finalizing the transaction with the travel agency turned out to be a warning of a major heart attack. At midnight, as the symptoms increased, I frantically telephoned for an ambulance, since Jim could no longer use a phone or remember my name.

He was taken straight into care, the authorities placing him into one of their old folks' retirement homes. Within the couple of months it took me to recover sufficiently to bring him home, he had lost many of his faculties through lack of professional care. While the staff had the experience of dealing with dementia in older people, they had found Jim too challenging, so that their care was both unsuitable and haphazard. When he came back to me, he was utterly confused and could no longer shower and shave alone. He needed strict supervision or he would use the wrong toiletries, rubbing toothpaste in his hair or cleaning his teeth with anything that lurked in a tube.

My patience wore thin. Not only was I still recovering from the heart attack, I now had the discomfort of angina, and Jim was also becoming increasingly aggressive. I only needed to say, "But you can't use shampoo for a mouthwash," and he'd lose his temper. Unfortunately, Jim was strong and fit enough to pack a punch. I found this new turn of events shattering, not only because of the danger, but because he had always been a most tender person and such a gentleman.

It is five years since I gave up caring for Jim. He was in the hospital for a long while, but since he no longer needed the level of care he had been receiving on the psychiatric ward, he was transferred to a care facility that I chose with great consideration. It's a lovely place with an outstanding staff, a gorgeous ambiance and delicious food. I visit him all the time to feed him, talk to him, and spread our photo album across his knees in the hope he might recognize some part of our life together. I get no response, but that's not important to me any more. My greatest wish is that perhaps he senses I'm there for him. For myself I'm making the most of what time we have, which might only be a matter of months.

I was told he has terminal cancer. This wasn't something I had ever considered, there being no instance of the disease in his background. At first it knocked me sideways, the knowledge that he is actually going to die.

As I contemplate the final journey we have to face before we go our separate ways, I realize how much it has changed me. It has given me the most prized asset that could be bestowed on any dementia caregiver: the ability to cope in the face of adversity and come out on the other side a stronger and wiser human being.

The writer lives in northwest England and has been writing since the age of seven. She has published on a wide variety of subjects, including outdoor pursuits, humor and local history. In 2005 one of her essays was included in the anthology *Stories of Strength*.

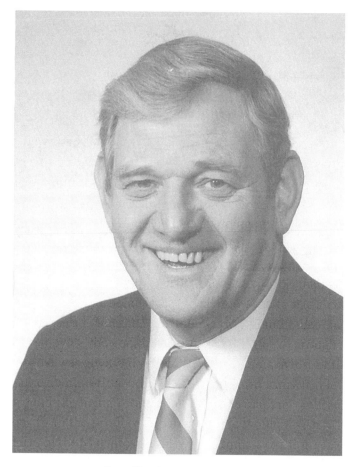

Tony Van Ingen, page 115

Behind Lace Curtains

Kali J. Van Baale

I sit before a pile of his denim overalls and white underwear, labeling the tags with his initials in black marker like I did for my children when they started school. Two small boxes containing family photos, hygiene items, and a faded crocheted afghan I made decades ago are next to the door, ready to be loaded. Two boxes are all he is allowed to take. I move a sack of his shoes as he stumbles into the room; slippers on the wrong feet even though I taped a large L and R on the top of each one, and I see that the fly of his overalls is open.

"Here, let me help you," I offer, tugging at the metal zipper.

"I love you," he repeats over and over.

"Yes, yes," I say, ever conscious of the time. "We've lost your glasses. Where did you put your glasses?"

Another search begins—under furniture, in closets, on top of cabinets. I check my watch and rub my swollen fingertips which protrude from the end of a dirty white cast on my wrist. During my search, I find that his T-shirt is in the toilet, the remote control is in the microwave oven, and he has poured his morning coffee into the sugar bowl. But no glasses.

"You're sore at me," he says.

"No. I'm not."

"You were sore at me yesterday."

"Yes, yesterday."

"I wet my pants."

"Yes, yesterday."

"I love you," he repeats. "I love you."

"Yes, yes, we're in a hurry." I softly shoo him away. "Now where are your glasses? We can't leave without your glasses."

He sags into his vinyl recliner with a whoosh of air under his weight and dozes off. His favorite recliner, I think—too big for his new room.

There is a pinch between my shoulder blades as I move the kitchen chairs back to the table out of the corner where he has pushed them. I am tired, but there is more to be done. I go to the window and press my forehead to the chilled pane, watch a cardinal eat from my birdfeeder in the backyard. I am wasting time, I know, but cannot help myself. I miss my garden, now overgrown and choked with foxtail and creeping Charlie, the corn patch ravaged by raccoons. I can't deny that my kitchen is also a mess. I see the piles of dirty pots and pans and know that the air in the room is stale. I don't notice so much anymore, but my children have made comments. Our dishwasher has not been fixed since his fall and it is difficult for me to wash the dishes by hand, which I explained to them, to no avail. These days, I am always falling behind. I keep reminding myself of this as I pack his boxes.

"He didn't push me," I had assured my son. "I was trying to catch him. He lost his balance is all. My fault really."

Ridiculous notion, I know, for a woman my age to think she could catch a grown man. Look at the result—both tumbling on top of the opened dishwasher door and me breaking my wrist instead of breaking our fall. There we lay, nearly six hours before my grandson found us, a jumbled pile of old bones on the floor.

"It's too dangerous," my son told me at the hospital. "You can't do this by yourself anymore. We'll get him the care he needs. You can visit any day of the week."

"Yes, yes, I know," I said. And I do know. His disease, his frightening journey of forgetfulness, cannot be helped by my poor eyesight, my bad heart, my brittle bones or paper-thin skin. Even though I know, still...

I pull the long drapes aside and there they are, his glasses, resting neatly on the sill behind the lace curtains. I unfold the earpieces and wipe the smudged lenses on the bottom of my shirt. I gently place them back on his weathered face, now passive with sleep, and smooth down a few long, wispy white strands of his hair with the palm of my hand. He needs a trim. I've always given him his haircuts. I did it in our early years because we never had the money to pay a barber, then later, because he just liked for me to do it. It suddenly occurs to me that I could still do that for him—give him his regular haircuts. When I visit in a few days, I could bring my hair scissors and electric trimmer. He will sit still for me, always calmed by my touch. Yes, I can still do that for him. I am hopeful to think that perhaps there are moments left to be shared between us, no matter where, or small, or seemingly inconsequential, that I can look towards and wrap my hands about to protect and keep warm.

But for now, I've wasted time again and our time is almost out. I wipe my eyes and return to the stack of clothing, to the boxes where I carefully printed his name on the side, the name I have shared for over sixty years. I hurry to finish before my son arrives to pick us up.

Kali grew up on a dairy farm in rural Iowa. She is an alumnus of Upper Iowa University and lives outside Des Moines with her husband and two children. She is the recipient of the 2005 Fred Bonnie Memorial Award for Best First Novel for her work of fiction, *The Space Between*.

For the Love of Rose

Susan Melchione

"Sangue delle mie vene!" she called out. The others in the room sat in silence. *"Sangue del mio cuore!"* she called out again. You could hear a pin drop. Rose smiled as she translated the Italian phrases she had just spoken. "'Blood of my veins! Blood of my heart!' This is what my mother said to me as she smothered me with kisses every day."

Rose enjoys sharing her life stories with the other members of the early-stage Alzheimer's group here at the Neuwirth Memory Disorders program at the Zucker Hillside Hospital Geriatric Center. Many of her long-term memories are joyful. Rose was one of five children born to immigrant parents. They were poor, but no one knew it. Her mother was a dressmaker. For a nickel's worth of material, she said, her mother made her the best dressed girl in school.

One day, while Rose was working with four hundred girls at a brassiere factory, a handsome man asked her where she went for lunch. She had no idea that he was about to become the love of her life. From that day on, Bert sat next to her at lunch and would not leave her side. In 1944, Bert proposed. Rose told her very religious Catholic mother about her engagement to this Jewish man. Without hesitation, her mother asked, *"Tu l'ami?"* which means

"Do you love him?" Rose responded, "Yes, I do!" and her mother took her in her arms and kissed her. Her mother knew that love transcends all.

Bert's love for Rose ran deep. After graduating high school in 1936, Bert had dreams of becoming a veterinarian. He was unable to complete his college education since his parents could not afford the $30 monthly tuition. Bert worked in his father's deli in Brooklyn until his aunt got him a job as a mechanic's helper, also in a brassiere factory. Bert was grateful for the $15 per week salary. He wanted to learn the trade, but the head mechanic would not teach him. Always believing that there is a solution to any problem, Bert became friendly with the factory foreman, who allowed Bert to stay at night so that he could teach himself about the machines. His diligence paid off. Eventually, they fired the head mechanic and replaced him with Bert.

He also worked hard doing free-lance work in the industrial sewing machine business and was proud to support himself and his lovely bride. When his father became ill, his mother suffered a nervous breakdown and his brother lost his job, Bert supported them all.

Bert and Rose thrived. They had a romantic relationship and they treasured their sons, whom they call their two "jewels." Over the years, Bert developed health problems, including heart problems, emphysema, and prostate cancer. Bert continues to use oxygen at all times and suffers from angina. Rose has suffered for many years with Crohn's Disease. Despite this, they managed to enjoy life.

Bert says that he lives by the motto "*A bi m'lacht*" which is Yiddish for "as long as you can laugh." Bert found it much more difficult to laugh after Rose developed symptoms of Alzheimer's Disease in 2002. He could not accept that Rose had an incurable disease. After all, he's the fix-it guy.

Bert had always believed in non-traditional solutions. He sub-scribed to several alternative medicine journals, all of which agreed that phosphatydylserine (PS), a nutrient, aided the memory, so he started Rose on PS. Looking for further assistance, Bert brought Rose to the Zucker Hillside Hospital Geriatric Center, but resisted the idea that the available medications may only slow the disease. Not good enough!

When I met Rose and Bert at the Geriatric Center, I immediately saw the emotional pain they were suffering as well as the power-ful connection between them. I personally provided support and education, and I encouraged their involvement in groups. In my experience, connecting with others who are also dealing with Alzheimer's Disease decreases isolation and enhances coping skills for both the person with the disease and his or her family. Rose, well aware of her memory deficits and saddened by her limita-tions, joined the early-stage Alzheimer's group. She was amazed by her memory of details of events in her life from long ago. She shared stories from her childhood, her work as a medical secre-tary, and even recited the preamble to the Constitution. She recalled how, as a child, she shared a bedroom with her grand-mother, whom she believes also had dementia. Her grandmother whispered the prayers of the rosary in bed. The sound of her prayers was comforting, and Rose would fall asleep to this sound.

Despite the frustration of her short-term memory loss, she remains inquisitive about life. Rose is still the Rose she has always been, except that her memory is failing and she must depend more on others. She can no longer drive and, as Bert discovered, can no longer be in a store alone. In 2005, Bert went to the pharmacy to pick up their medicine while Rose looked in another store for a crossword puzzle book. Bert waited outside the store, assuming that Rose was browsing (Rose certainly looks the same, and it's common for a loved one to forget that the brain is not function-ing as it did before.) When Rose did not appear, Bert panicked. She was nowhere to be found. Bert was concerned that even if a kind person found her, Rose would likely give a home address from long ago. Bert called his son, considered calling the police, and circled the area in his car for over an hour. He finally found Rose five blocks away, walking on a major road.

Now she is never out of his sight. Whenever I go to the waiting room to escort Rose and the other members to the group room, Bert asks, "Can I come in?" At first, I explained that the group is only for those with the memory problem. It gives them the freedom to express whatever they need to without concern about their loved one's response. Bert understood. It doesn't stop him, however, from asking every time, "Can I come in?" Now I just say "no" with a smile, and we laugh. He says with a grin, "You can't blame me for trying," and I certainly don't.

Acknowledging his need for support, Bert participates in the caregiver support group. Bert told the group that he stays up at night trying to invent a cure for dementia. He pressures himself and shares this feeling by asking me, "So, have you found a cure yet?" Everyone in the group knows there is none yet, but each one still longs to hear the answer "Yes!" We discuss the research that's currently taking place. But that's not good enough for Bert. He says, "I know there's a cure. I just have to find it."

Bert takes his responsibility to care for Rose seriously. He does admit to being human and sometimes his patience is exhausted by her repetitive questions. For the first several repetitions, Bert answers calmly, but admits to sometimes raising his voice and saying, "You asked me that already." He then experiences feelings of guilt. Rose doesn't remember. It's not her fault. It's the disease. He knows that. The caregiver group members empathize with him. They know what it feels like to love someone and hate the disease that he or she has.

The group members recommend other outlets. These include redirecting her, going into another room, calling a friend, or taking more time alone to recharge. Bert listens, but having more time away from Rose is not his preference. With a great deal of encouragement, Bert allowed Rose to go to an adult day program. At the end of the day, she doesn't remember the activities, but like many with this disease, she remembers the feelings and knows that she had fun. The group members encouraged Bert to increase Rose's attendance at the program, so that he could have more time for himself. Bert, who has spent the past 62 years with Rose, replied, "But what would I do with myself?"

Bert also expresses frustration about Rose moving his papers. He puts something down, and when he looks again, it's not there. He realizes that it's foolish to ask Rose where she put it because she can't remember. He asks her anyway. She says, "I don't remember," and he replies, "It must be the night shift," and begins searching. The important papers are the most upsetting to lose. So I asked Bert if he could put them in a locked drawer or in drawers that Rose does not go through. Bert replied, "She enjoys going through my drawers!" and they both laughed. Rose responded with a sparkle in her eye, "It's true!"

How they love each other. When Bert needed to leave the house for work, he would kiss tissues, and leave each one beautifully folded on the nightstands of his wife and sons' beds so that they would always have his kiss with them. Bert said, "If I could take all of the love songs in the world and condense them into one, that would show the way we feel about one another."

"I love him so much," Rose says.

"You'll get over it!" Bert jokes. They both laugh. A minute later, I start to ask Rose a question. Forgetting that she just told me her feelings, she interrupts and says, "Do you want to know if I love him?"

"Yes," I reply.

"I do...he's my heartbeat."

"Then she'd better take a nitro!" Bert says. *A bi m'lacht*...they have found a way to laugh again.

Bert is a hero. He has the mind of an engineer and a heart of gold. He would do anything for anyone. But this Mr. Fix-It, with all the love in the world, cannot fix this. What he can do is laugh, and care for his bride. And truly everything he does is for the love of Rose.

With gratitude to Rose and Bert Baron for sharing their story and loving energy.

Susan Melchione is a Licensed Clinical Social Worker and Program Coordinator of the Neuwirth Memory Disorder Program of the Zucker Hillside Hospital Geriatric Center. She holds a Master of Social Work degree from Adelphi University. For the past 15 years, she has been a direct-care provider to adults and families with neurological disorders, with a specialty in geriatrics.

Teacher's Pet

Sandy McPherson Carrubba

My husband Joe always made life interesting, with his quirky sense of humor and funny antics. But one summer his behavior took a strange turn. He grabbed items from the back of the refrigerator without moving those in front of what he wanted, so I was constantly mopping up the spills and messes that he caused. After more than 38 years of marriage, I knew it was not normal when he ran outside early one morning in his pajamas, claiming he was looking for something. I sought a reason for his illogical and puzzling behavior. An emergency appointment with his neurologist provided the troubling answer: Joe had Alzheimer's.

After hearing what the doctor said, Joe referred to himself as "This stupid old *B&%#*#!" "Don't talk like that about the man I love," I'd tell him. But he'd repeat the expression whenever he became exasperated with himself, which happened more and more as time went on. We didn't like the diagnosis, but we could not change it: we were in this boat and had to row. If we worked together, I knew we could steer through the shoals. The challenge was to figure out how to get Joe to grab an oar and work with me. I didn't want him to give up.

The doctor told us that Joe was right on the edge, between the mild and moderate stages of the disease. The doctor prescribed a medication and assured me it would make Joe like he was two years before. He didn't tell me it would take three months to see positive effects from the medicine. Within a week of the diagnosis, I felt as if I had already lost my spouse. His voice became flat and expressionless. He no longer laughed, even when I teased him or told a joke.

Joe had already overcome many obstacles. In 1999 he was diagnosed with aggressive prostate cancer. Six years earlier he had suffered a heart attack. The summer before the Alzheimer's diagnosis, he had his second stroke. I often referred to him as "the Energizer Bunny," because he kept on going. However, the latest diagnosis seemed to take away his will to endure.

I wanted my husband back from the despair into which he had fallen. I refused to wait helplessly for each stage of the illness to take place. I sat Joe down and said, "You're still Joe and I'm still Sandy, and we're still together. We are going to walk forward, together, as far as we can go." He cried and hugged me. He nodded in agreement, but I doubted he understood.

What could I do to keep him with me? I felt as if I had been thrown into deep water and was trying to keep my head above the waves. We faced many uncertainties. No one, not even the doctor, could tell me how long Joe would continue to dress, toilet, or bathe himself, but we could appreciate the things we had always done together. We still enjoyed walks by the river, going for ice cream or having dinner with a few friends.

The constant tension of supervising him, to keep him safe from himself exhausted me. Too much stimulation exhausted him, I found, so I limited the number of visitors at any one time. He couldn't remember to take his pills unless I reminded him. I solved that problem with a container that had separate boxes for morning, noon, evening, and bedtime pills. He rushed up or down staircases, tripped and bumped himself. He bent down to retrieve an item from the floor and forgot he was under the table, so he cut his head open. Each day, his skin showed more rainbow colors of bruises. I feared someone might think I abused him. I remained watchful and constantly reminded him to hold the handrail on the stairway. "*Be careful,*" became my motto.

My stomach often rebelled because of the tension. I was already tired when I awoke in the morning. I knew we couldn't go on this way or I wouldn't be able to care for myself, let alone my ailing husband. It was as if I was trying to outrun a storm and I'd become too winded to continue. "Take care of yourself," his doctor told me. Others did as well. I wondered just how to accomplish this when I had to look out for Joe. Our grown daughters lived across the country from us and seldom visited. My life had changed dramatically. Ordinarily, Joe would have fixed a leaking pipe or checked the windshield wiper fluid in the car. Now I had to have a plumber or mechanic do tasks for me that I couldn't do myself.

Still, parts of our former life could be salvaged. Joe thought he had to give up everything. I reassured him that our life wasn't over. He ushered at church before his diagnosis; I suggested he continue. The other ushers supervised him and helped Joe still feel a part of services. At times when he looked confused, another usher guided him. They changed his assignment to a less busy part of the church. Men from one of his organizations picked him up and took him to club meetings. His older brother began taking him out for lunch occasionally. Little by little he grew more animated. We continued attending classical music concerts and a local live theater. Dramas became difficult for him to follow; Joe enjoyed the musicals much more.

Some evenings when he had trouble reading and concentrating, he sat near our stereo and played big band music. That relaxed him. I often heard him singing along with a vocalist. Sometimes I asked him to dance, which made him grin. I liked the closeness and basked in it.

As the first autumn after his diagnosis progressed, I worried about how to keep Joe busy and stimulated through the winter. He worked in the garden when weather permitted. It took him two weeks to trim back our roses, but after he finished he felt a sense of accomplishment. In our area of the northeast, we don't garden in the winter; Joe needed other activities to keep him involved, since his club meetings were held only once a month. He took no interest in the puzzles we bought. I needed to solve the puzzle of how to keep him stimulated and active.

I needed a break from my continuous "guard duty". His neurologist had stressed with me to never leave Joe alone, yet I was reluctant to entrust him to someone else's care. If he simply sat at home, he would become bored. He couldn't do involved projects alone or use power tools without supervision. I encouraged him to make the statues he once made for family members. Despite my urging, he never did begin another.

Finally, I looked up adult daycare facilities to see if anything was available near us. I made it clear to Joe that he didn't have a choice of whether to attend, but he could pick the facility he preferred. I explained that I needed time for myself one day a week, and that he must be in a safe place. I made an appointment for Joe to try a daycare center for four hours. I inspected it and found that it did not offer very much; it reminded me of a warehouse, everyone just sitting around, purposeless. Perhaps I was expecting more than daycare could give us. Although we both felt discouraged by that first experience, we didn't give up.

I liked the second facility's bright and cheery atmosphere. It had been suggested to us by a social worker from the local Alzheimer's Association. While there, Joe made a wreath and brought it home, but complained that most of the decorations were on it before he started, and anything he chose to add was glued on by a staff member. He felt he hadn't made the wreath at all, he told me. Obviously, his ability level hadn't been considered.

We tried a third facility. "This is the one I want," he said. "They don't treat everyone the same like the last one did." So Joe began attending adult social daycare once a week. I was amazed at the difference it made. By this time, his medication was taking effect, too. Since he was functioning at a higher level than some clients there, the staff assigned him tasks the others couldn't do. He helped chop vegetables and prepare the noon meals, with supervision. He helped decorate for holidays. The facility offered transportation. Some days I let staff pick him up and bring him home, so I had more time to myself. Other days I had him taken to daycare, but I picked him up. I liked the flexibility.

Joe liked the daycare. His self-confidence and self-esteem rose steadily. He came home enthused about his activities and told me about it whether I was ready to listen or not. "Guess what I did at daycare today?" he asked me. He looked forward to going and often asked, "Is tomorrow the day I go to daycare?"

The facility was small and intimate. With its stuffed chairs and recliners, it felt as if we walked into someone's home. The staff there seemed genuinely interested in each client and saw each one as an individual. Joe became a part of the place; he said it felt like a family to him. He was one of the more popular care recipients because he laughed and joked with the staff.

While he attended daycare, I joined a friend for lunch, scheduled my own doctor visits, or took a nap. By having time away from one another, we received needed stimulation and gained a new perspective. Joe's laugh rang through the house once again as our cat amused him or he read a joke. When I teased him, he guffawed. His laugh sounded like music to me; I hadn't heard it for so long and missed it terribly. Once he started daycare, he stopped calling himself derogatory names. The daycare experience helped him recognize he still had worth and purpose.

At his appointment with his neurologist, he bragged to the doctor that he was "teacher's pet" at daycare. The doctor grinned and asked him about that. Joe excitedly told about all the assignments he got that others did not. He said he knew everyone there loved him. He told his siblings about his being "teacher's pet" as well. I don't know if they realized how important daycare had become for his well-being.

One day, when Joe seemed particularly lucid, I asked him why he enjoyed daycare so much. "I'm with people who are in the same boat as I am," he said. "We all have AD and know what each of us is going through. We understand each other in a way no else can. We don't have to explain anything to each other." I smiled and reminded him that he had given me a hard time about attending. "Now you know why I wanted you to go," I said. He thanked me and told me he realized what it did for him.

I liked the change in him. I felt as if I greeted my husband on his return from a trip. That's the best part: I got my husband back for a while. That was enough to prepare us for a long boat ride through calm or stormy waters.

A graduate of the State University of New York at Oswego, Sandy's writing career spans fifty years. A mother of two, she is active in church and environmental causes.

Part III
THE GRANDPARENTS

What families have in common the world around is that they are the place where people learn who they are and how to be that way.

—Jean Illsley Clarke

Wherever He Goes,
I Will Follow

Amy Shore

It took thirteen months to adopt my younger daughter Lucy and, during the adoption, my grandfather's health took a nosedive. The heart can be pulled in so many different directions all at once. But through all this, one thing was constant: my heart was full of love.

It all began with an alarming phone call from my mother in Florida. She and Dad had retired to a condominium there, full of sunshine and golden life, leaving behind the cold, snowy winters of Massachusetts. However, they stayed anchored to the Bay State by my father's parents, lifelong New Englanders in their eighties who could not fathom leaving "home."

"Zadie had a fall," my mother told me as gently as she could, knowing that her words would immediately cause alarm bells to clang in my head. My mother was sugar-coating it. My father told me the whole story. Zadie, My grandfather, had driven my grandmother to a doctor's appointment. Not wanting his elderly wife to walk on the snow and ice, he let her off at the front door to the doctor's office, then drove to the back parking lot, planning to join her in the waiting room. He never arrived.

My grandmother, at first annoyed that her husband of sixty years was taking so long, stuck her head outside the door, to see him lying prone on the cold, icy asphalt. Paramedics revived him and he was whisked to the hospital, where it was later determined that he had suffered a stroke.

That was his last day of freedom as an independent adult. No one knew then that my grandfather, the person who loved to go to the grocery store and take his time selecting the best cuts of meat; the person who once literally took the shirt off his back when I mentioned that it would make a great beach cover-up; the person who loved to pore over the morning newspaper and watch *Jeopardy* on a little black and white TV at the kitchen table so that my grandmother could watch her soaps in comfort and in color, was never coming home again.

Directly from his stay at the hospital, he became a resident at a nearby nursing home. My grandmother was worried. She was unable to care for him the way he needed, and my grandfather needed a lot of care: the stroke had robbed him of his ability to walk or to use his right arm and hand. At first we all thought that intense physical therapy would help him shape up and go home, but the doctors soon confirmed what we had suspected for several months: my grandfather was also suffering from dementia.

On my first visit to see him at the nursing home, I saw my once powerful and nimble Zadie imprisoned in a wheelchair. Always a capable, active man, he hated being stuck in a chair. While my grandmother and parents talked in the corner of the room with the physical therapist, my grandfather, in his wheelchair next to the floral sofa on which I sat, attempted to escape. He used his good arm and hand to move his legs and, ingeniously, he moved himself onto the sofa. I watched, incredulous yet proud of his determination, but the alarm on his wheelchair sounded, alerting the staff. They stepped in and put him back in the chair, this time with a seat belt. He hated that chair.

The next time I visited Zadie, he was walking with a walker. The wheelchair was history. When he saw me, his oldest grandchild, he instinctively reached into his pocket, looking for a single dollar bill. Throughout my childhood, my Zadie always gave me a dollar bill; he called himself "the dollar Zadie." It gave him such pleasure to give all of us little ones a dollar, to see our faces brighten and react as if we had won the lottery. It didn't matter that now I was in my late thirties and a parent myself; I was his Amy and he was my Zadie.

Instead of a dollar, out came some folded paper notes. He seemed confused and upset that he couldn't remember what he was looking for. I asked my grandmother what the notes were, and she showed me: one had my grandfather's name written in bold, "LEO SHORE." Another had his room number printed in big, bold numbers. The last was my grandmother's name and telephone number, a number that I committed to memory at age five and had been Zadie's telephone number for more than fifty years. He was obsessively afraid that he would forget who he was, where he was and how to contact his wife, the only person he completely trusted now that his mind was dissolving.

I lived out of state but my father and grandmother kept me informed about my grandfather's scuffles at the nursing home. Awakening in the middle of the night, forgetting where he was and why he was there, he punched orderlies who tried to calm him. Another scuffle occurred in the shower stall, when a male nurse attempted to help my grandfather wash. Paranoid, he refused any medication, accusing the nurses of trying to poison him. The nursing staff warned my grandmother that if he continued to be combative, he would not be able to stay there. But where would he go? There were very few nursing homes that had a bed open for a man with Alzheimer's Disease. Instead, he was drugged every day to keep him calm and serene.

Finally, I was able to fulfill a promise I made to my Zadie thirteen months earlier. One cold, snowy December afternoon in

Massachusetts, reminiscent of the day of my grandfather's stroke, I walked into the nursing home with my family: my husband Dave, my eleven year old daughter Miranda, and the newest addition to the family, our one year old daughter Lucy. I knew where to find my grandfather; he would be upstairs in the day room where the TV was on but no one was watching. Typically, my grandmother would be with me when I visited Zadie, but a fall in the bathroom had caused her a brief stay in the hospital. This time I would be on my own. I told myself to be ready for anything. Without my grandmother, would he recognize me? What would we talk about? Was this going to be one of his good days?

We entered the lobby. Miranda walked briskly around the corner to the elevator and pushed the buttons; she had been here several times before and assumed that this was just a home away from home. I held my little one in my arms; her big dark eyes drank in the scenery. My husband was the first to see my grandfather and pointed me in his direction.

There he was in the hallway, slumped in a chair, surrounded by other nursing home residents, most of them with their eyes closed, sound asleep. I knew in my heart that this was most likely what he did most of the time when no one was visiting him: he slept the end of his life away alone with his dreams, what he remembered.

I gently touched my Zadie's soft, wrinkled hand, the hand that held mine countless times when he brought me as a young girl to the penny candy store to fill a brown bag full of dots, chocolate coins, bubble gum cigars, and licorice whips. That same hand around my waist as I clung to his stocky neck, afraid of the sound of the cannon at the local parade that he loved to take me to each year. My protector, my provider. His eyes fluttered open and he looked straight into my face.

"Hello," he said, rubbing his eyes, trying to wake up and figure out what was going on.

"Hi, Zadie!" I said, cheerfully, smiling at my grandfather. "How are you?"

"Amy," he said, seeking confirmation. Time was now difficult for my grandfather to comprehend. In his foggy mind, a visit we had made six months ago to him occurred just yesterday. But there was that smile, helping him to resemble the grandfather I have always known. His eyes were so expressive, filled with love in remembering me.

"Let's go to my room," he said, slowly standing up and shuffling down the hall. I was on one side of him, Miranda on the other, Dave and the baby were behind. For Zadie's benefit we moved at a snail's pace, pretending that this was always the way we walked. I smiled at the men and women we passed, most of them in wheelchairs or with walkers, wishing they too had visitors. It was apparent from the way they looked at us that there was a real hunger for visitors from the outside world, especially children.

We five huddled into my grandfather's small, twin-bedded room, the fourth or fifth he'd had in two years (my grandfather argued with roommates—a territorial thing. The staff tried to keep my grandfather living alone when it was possible.) In the nursing home there was always shuffling and change, ironic since those with memory deficiencies function best with quiet and stability.

"Zadie, I want you to meet my daughter Lucy. We just brought her home from Guatemala. Do you remember me telling you we were adopting a baby?"

"Yes," he said, focusing his entire being on my little one. She looked intently at my grandfather. My past, my present, and my future all intermingled at that moment. Last year, I wasn't sure this moment would ever come; I willed my grandfather to be well enough to introduce him to his newest great-granddaughter. Selfishly, I wanted that moment. Throughout my life, my grandfather was always there: he kvelled at my Bat Mitzvah, patiently taught me how to drive when my own father hadn't the patience, watched me graduate from high school and then college, danced at my wedding and shared in the joy when my daughter was born, making him a great grandpa. Regardless of the circumstances, he was always beaming with pride and offering wisdom, even when I didn't ask for it. I couldn't imagine him not being a part of our most recent joy, so I brought our joy to him.

"Helloooo," he said in his sing-song Zadie voice, patting the spot near him on the bed for my Lucy to sit. My one year old clung to me fervently, but she didn't cry. I sat next to Zadie and Lucy sat on my lap, never taking her eyes off the man who was smiling at her. With his weathered, wrinkled white fingers he gently touched the velvet brown skin on the back of Lucy's little hand. "Helloooo," he repeated. "I'm your Zadie!"

"I've got something for you," he said, standing up and moving to the bedside table. He opened the drawer and took out a bag of cookies, the kind you buy at 7-Eleven that come two to a package. He handed them to my Lucy, who didn't move a muscle. I took them, opened the plastic wrap, and because Lucy was too little to eat a cookie, I took a bite instead. Miranda ate another. My grandfather chuckled, seeing us enjoying the cookies—a gift from Zadie. Throughout my life my Zadie was always trying to feed his visitors. Most of the time it was an elaborate fruit bowl that he designed himself. He would walk around the living room, offering paper napkins and beautiful selections from the produce department. He would lavish praise on the redness of the Macintosh apples, the firmness of the green grapes, the sweetness of the cantaloupe slices. He always wanted to please his guests. He was always thinking of others. Nothing had changed. The nurses complained that my grandfather hid food in his room in the strangest of places. Perhaps he was planning for this very moment when he would be "entertaining" again.

I looked closely at my grandfather. He wore brown polyester slacks and not one but three pullover knit shirts. Most days, he forgot that he was already wearing a shirt, so he put on another. Over his shirts, he wore a cardigan sweater, the kind Mr. Rogers made famous on TV. On his feet were Velcro-fastened sneakers, similar to the ones my Lucy was wearing on her little feet. He was shorter than I remembered from my last visit, now the same height as my eleven year old. His once dark, wavy hair was now pure white. Sometimes on his face there crept a vacant look which would startle me. But something always brought him back to me—that twinkle in his eye or the smile on his face—to show he wasn't too far away.

After a short visit, we told Zadie it was time for us to go. He asked me where Lil was. It was the first time he called my Nana by her first name to me. I told him that she was recuperating in the hospital after a fall, that he talked with her this morning on the telephone at the nurse's station. He'd forgotten. "That's right," he said softly, trying to remember.

"Who ya got there, Leo?" asked one of the nurses, a big smile on her face when she saw my grandfather slowly making his way down the hallway, surrounded by his "groupies."

"This is my daughta, my son-in-law, and their daughtas — my granddaughtas," he gushed with his Massachusetts accent. He introduced us to his "special friend" as he called her. I corrected my Zadie: I was his oldest granddaughter, this was my husband, and these girls were his great granddaughters. But I could tell it didn't matter much. Love is love is love, and who really cared by which degree it existed?

Passing Lucy to my husband as we neared the elevator, I turned and gave my grandfather a big hug. His body was soft to the touch, not frail but old. Whenever I said goodbye, I didn't know if it was for the final time. "I love you, Zadie! You take good care of yourself! I'll see you soon!" I said through tears in my eyes.

"Ba-bye!" he waved, his smile still painted on his face as the elevator doors closed. "See ya tomorrow!"

I knew that the next time I saw him he wouldn't remember our visit. Yet my Zadie will always be my Zadie. It's just that now he is in transition. My motherly instincts help me know how to love him now that we have, in a sense, reversed roles. He was always there for me, and now I am there for him. Wherever he goes, I will follow.

Amy Shore is the author of two books: *Waiting for Lucinda* and *High School Hall Pass*. She is a former high school English teacher who taught for 13 years in both public and private schools throughout the United States. A freelance writer and newspaper columnist, Amy's essays have appeared in a variety of anthologies, journals and magazines and she is an editor of this book. She lives in Houston, Texas with her husband and two daughters.

Love, the Greatest Gift of All

Julie Sieving

Entering the nursing home, I was overcome by a wave of emotions. As my four-year old niece, Chelsea and I anxiously made our way towards my grandparents' room, I wondered what we would encounter. Both of my grandparents have been residents here for about two years. Grandpa is bedridden and completely immobile, but he still understands some of what goes on around him. Grandma's condition is the opposite: she is in good physical condition, but Alzheimer's Disease has rendered her mentally incompetent. She used to have quite a few good moments. Now that her disease has progressed, her mind appears to be in constant turmoil.

We reached their room and I hesitated momentarily before peeking in to see if Grandma was there. I found her standing at the head of Grandpa's bed, caressing his cheek and forehead. As she turned to me, I could see tears of despair trickling down her grief-stricken face. I tried to act cheerful and said, "Happy birthday, Grandma! You shouldn't be crying on your birthday!"

"Oh yeah! I guess so," she said, with a confused look.

"Did you get a birthday cake?"

"I don't know... Yes!" she said, as she walked over to the door, where there was tacked up a birthday banner with her name on it.

She thought it was a cake. A moment later she spotted Chelsea. "Ain't he cute?" She asked, pointing to Chelsea. Then she walked back over to my grandpa and became all teary-eyed again.

Looking for a way to draw her attention away from him, I said, "Come sit down over here so we can visit."

She nodded yes, as if she understood, but instead, she walked over to the window. She pointed out across the parking lot and said, "Black things to roam forever but nobody around to see them. Everything that happens; see out there." Then the tears came rolling down her face again. All of sudden, a smile spread across her face as Chelsea caught her attention again. "She's so sweet. I love you."

I tried to think of something cheerful to talk about. I told her about my writing assignment for my college class and asked her if I could write about her. She paused as if thinking about it. "That would be nice. I love you. Ain't they cute?" she asked once again as she looked in Chelsea's direction. Pointing to Grandpa, she said, "See her shirt and everything." This started her crying again.

I decided that it might be good for Grandma if I took her away for a little while. I tried to reassure her. "Grandpa will be okay." I said. "The nurses will take care of him while you are gone." As Chelsea and I led Grandma from the room, I noticed that she was wiping her tears with a rubber glove. I wanted to laugh, yet I felt so sad. This person I loved was so helpless. Without too much fuss, I exchanged the glove for a tissue.

We arrived at a small local restaurant a short time later. "What would you like for dinner, Grandma?"

"I don't care. I'm here." She looked at me with tears in her eyes. "I love you!"

I ordered her a hamburger, shake, and fries. She couldn't remember how to use a straw. She tried to drink out of the plastic lid and tried eating her catsup plain by scooping it up on her finger. Otherwise, the meal was pretty uneventful.

Getting her back into the car was another story. I opened her door. "We are going to go now," I said.

She nodded, "OK."

"We need to get in the car."

"OK," but she didn't comprehend and she didn't move.

"Sit right here!" I said as I patted the seat.

'Sometimes there's not very much to do that because there is cars," she said as she finally climbed into the front seat.

As I was driving, Grandma overheard Chelsea tell me that she loved me.

Grandma said, "Thank you! That really helps me good."

I could see that Grandma was getting tired, so I drove her back to the home. I took her back to her room, told her goodbye and that I loved her and gave her a hug. She said she loved me too. As I waited for the elevator door to open, I spotted Grandma in the hallway, walking towards me. I smiled at her, but she didn't recognize me.

Even though Grandma no longer knows me, she still loves me. She loves everybody. She stands over my grandpa's bed for hours, just watching over him. She no longer knows that he is her husband, just someone that she loves very deeply. The nursing home tried to separate them, but she always searched until she found *that man* again.

In one moment her mind can't comprehend even the simplest of ideas, in the next instant, she'll stop and look at me and say, "I love you!" She says this with the most truthful, loving expression on her face. I have always known that her love for me is forever engraved on her heart. In all her confusion, Grandma can still give and receive the greatest gift of all.

_____

The writer lives and works in Ohio with her husband and two children. She is a graduate of Terra State University.

Bridging Fact and Perception

Lyn Michaud

Alzheimer's Disease defies the unspoken rules of communication. We are willing to perpetuate myths with children: Santa Claus, the Easter Bunny, superheroes and fairy princesses. Long after the truth is revealed, we continue to tell these little white lies because they create a connection between us. When dealing with older parents and grandparents, however, we correct their memory errors and expect them to stay with us in our reality.

The situation creates a moral dilemma—do we correct inaccuracies to maintain strict truth, or allow the people we love to find happiness in altered memories? Reminding an Alzheimer's patient of her former knowledge or teaching memory skills can't remedy the physical deterioration or the behavioral symptoms caused by the disease. The behaviors that seem inappropriate are not learned, but the result of a physical condition. Alzheimer's Disease isn't as yet something a person can be healed from, like a broken bone.

When my paternal grandfather was diagnosed with Alzheimer's, it was considered a severe form of memory loss. Doctors speculated this form of dementia skipped a generation. Knowing that I could be the next in line to develop Alzheimer's became a driving force to make me think about how I would like to be treated were it to strike me.

Once, my grandfather reported his wife missing to the police. They called off the search after contacting one of his sons, who informed them that my grandfather's wife had died a few years before. I knew how much my grandfather loved my grandmother and how much he missed her. I recall thinking that if I loved someone, I wouldn't want to be reminded over and over of my loss.

He was no longer able to live alone and was admitted to an assisted living facility. While there, he nailed his door shut to prevent the nurses from entering his room. We assumed the routine care felt like an intrusion.

Despite this first experience with my grandfather, I was no more prepared when my independent and spirited maternal grandmother was diagnosed with Alzheimer's. I enjoyed visiting my grandmother with my infant daughter, and she developed an affection for my husband. On one visit, she expected my husband's customary hug. He'd grown a beard for the winter and his whiskers tickled her face; she stopped, looked at his beard, and reached up to touch it with a look of awe like a child discovering something wonderful for the first time.

"Is it warm?" she asked.

"Keeps my face warm all winter, especially when I go out in the cold."

My grandmother hugged herself and pretended to shiver. "I'd like to grow one over my whole body."

We all laughed, but I accepted her wish as perfect logic: if the need arose perhaps bodies would adapt a different hair pattern growth. I didn't and still don't consider her thoughts inappropriate nor a sign of the beginning stage of Alzheimer's Disease; they showed creative thinking.

As the disease progressed, our personal connection slipped; she would call me by the wrong name or remember me in another time with another relationship. I struggled between not wanting to hurt her feelings and my need for personal acknowledgment. I wanted the person I'd become to be recognized.

My mother intervened with facts when her mother first began living in memories. After my grandmother sold the farm and moved to a new apartment in a retirement community, I visited her. My mother went with me to show me around and introduce me to the staff. We toured the apartment and stopped in the bathroom. My mother pointed to a safety bench in the shower and told me who brought it. My grandmother spoke up.

"Edwin brought it." My grandmother was pleased. "He's so good to me."

Edwin was my grandfather, who had been gone for over 20 years. My mother was quick to correct her. "No, so and so brought it for you."

My grandmother looked doubtful, but didn't press the issue. I knew my grandfather hadn't brought the bench, and I also saw how believing he had made my grandmother feel special. My mother was a nurse for 40 years; she took care of hospitalized patients with various stages of dementia. I deferred to her experience but persisted in thinking that dreams brought happiness. If there was no harm done, I didn't see a problem in allowing fantasy instead of absolute truth.

Her disease caused a rapid decline. One winter day, she took a walk without a coat. A couple recognized her and stopped. She didn't know where she was going or where her home was. They knew, and returned her to her home. My family decided it was time for her to move to a nursing home. That decision causes conflicting feelings in me. I would like to see other options instead of removing older people from society. However, I do recognize the independence assisted living allows by relieving the person from feeling like a burden to family members.

Absence takes away the personal feelings Alzheimer's invokes. I moved across the country to attend graduate school. I admit it was easier for me with increased distance; I had a life of my own and my grandmother had people to love her and take care of her.

My mother kept me informed and sometimes called to consult with me about a medication or treatment. I stayed on top of new scientific developments and could explain to her the mechanism of action of medications or new developments in Alzheimer's research. When we discussed some of my grandmother's behaviors, I tended not to sympathize with how others perceived her actions. But I was concerned about how others' actions affected my grandmother. She became a patient to me; I could look at her disease from a clinical standpoint. I would in subtle ways try to get my mother to look at the events with emotional detachment. I played devil's advocate with other points of view—maybe my grandmother found happiness or comfort in her memories and wanted to stay that way.

During a visit to my parents, we went to the nursing home to see my grandmother. My mother told Gram Gram who I was and I thought I saw a flicker of recognition. If it wasn't recognition, my grandmother at least repeated my name and repeated back the facts of how we were related. In that moment, I realized I no longer cared if she knew me. I wanted her happy and let her be in charge of the conversation. I listened for clues and made silly comments. She laughed with me and I don't even know why. I just know we had a good time. What could I say? I wasn't my grandmother's caregiver and I didn't have to correct her. The experience was pretend; I could be the aunt who spoiled her niece and then sent her home to her parents.

My grandfather left me a legacy of Alzheimer's Disease. As a young mother I had to confront my fears that one day I may not recognize my child and not be in control of my own life. The inevitable seemed to loom. Would I want to be told the truth or be allowed to live in my fantasies? Logic would tell me that I would prefer to be told the truth, but with my brain ravaged by disease, logic isn't the only thing in play.

Instead of presuming Alzheimer's Disease might not be a possibility for me, I've thought about my future. I don't want to be forced to fight for my right to live in happy dreams. My daughter says I want to know everything about everything. The possibility of a breakdown in the pathway to my memories leads me to take advice from experts and do mental exercises. I've decided to plan ahead and put in writing how I want to be treated, a way of exercising my right to make decisions while I have time.

Living Wills address treatment options and how one wants to die. I want a similar plan to direct my quality of life, how I want to be treated in the event I develop Alzheimer's. I want my daughter and my caregivers to remember I'm captive in a world I no longer recognize. I don't want to be judged. I don't want to be told I'm wrong. I want to be accepted in my new persona. I want to be hugged instead of kept at an institutional distance because I don't live in reality. And if I mention someone I once knew and ask a question, find out what I want to know before insisting on telling me the truth. If I tell a story about my life and it doesn't seem true, let me have the final say. Let me remember and live in the happiest moments of my life and change the worst experiences to positive should-have-beens. Help me laugh. Common courtesy should prevail. Even if we believe a person is a crazy old coot, we need to remember to talk to him, tell him what we're doing, and treat him like an adult instead of a child.

After my grandmother passed on I wondered, had I been more involved would I have expected her to stay in touch with reality. I now volunteer with an organization whose mission is to encourage enjoyment in life. On Valentine's Day, we visited a nursing home to deliver valentine cards and entertain the residents. When our song leader asked for requests, the residents asked for patriotic songs and songs from the 1940's and earlier. One elderly lady sat through most of our visit in a quiet world of her own. Near the end of the singing, she whispered a request for a song we didn't remember well. She led us through the song, not skipping a word, her voice strong. She had tears in her eyes when we finished, whether for joy in her memories or sorrow for her loss, I didn't know and she never said. For her, the song provided a connection between the past and the present.

During that visit, I spent most of my time with a man who told me in detail about his wartime experiences and the places he'd lived as a civilian. I had lived in many of the same places and we had a good time talking about landmarks and discussing how things had changed. As I was leaving, one of the staff commented to me that I shouldn't believe a word he said; he wasn't in his right mind. I reviewed our conversation and decided it didn't matter if his memories were true. I listened to him and his eyes sparkled.

Even those of us who have experienced Alzheimer's Disease with family members can do no better than guess what it's like to have the disease. The patients are not like children; we have no control over their behavior or thoughts. A few simple measures help us maintain bonds. Before visiting we make peace with our feelings regarding the loss of the former relationship. We respect them. Mutual respect bridges reality, in fact or perception. We treat them the way we would want to be treated.

A resident of Colorado, Lyn Michaud holds a Bachelors Degree in biology and chemistry and was a member of the Weld County Board of Public Health and Environment. Her articles and stories have appeared in *Learning through History, Characters* and *Home Cooking*.

The Wedding Crasher

Penny Johnson Jerald

Like many families, mine has endured the suffering and loss caused by Alzheimer's Disease. Alzheimer's first invaded my family one day more than twenty years ago. It was a beautiful June afternoon. Everything was perfect. It was my wedding day.

But then I approached my grandmother, whom I hadn't seen during the years I was away at college. I looked forward to the warm, loving smile and smothering hug she always greeted us grandkids with. But this day, her look was different, kind of hazy. I asked her if she was still enjoying the sealskin coat and hat I'd sent her for her birthday. Not only did she not remember the coat... she didn't know who I was. At the time, I thought she was just getting old and was experiencing a little senility. It was easier to simply chalk it up to old age. I had no idea at the time how serious her condition was.

Over the next months, Grandma had several episodes of irrational behavior. There were times of extreme paranoia, loss of memory, disorientation; on one occasion, she set fire to my mom's kitchen. She was soon diagnosed with Alzheimer's Disease. After many failed attempts to keep her with family, she was placed in a nearby care facility. For fifteen years, my family watched helplessly as our sweet grandmother's mental and physical health deteriorated.

Grandma died at age 86, robbed of irreplaceable memories, a shadow of what she once was.

My prayer is that a cure will be found so that no one else will have to endure being robbed of themselves, and no other families will be deprived of their loved ones because of Alzheimer's Disease.

Penny Johnson Jerald won critical and popular acclaim for her guest starring role as the devious political wife in the first season of Fox's Emmy-nominated drama "24." She then returned to the show as a regular, stirring up more trouble as the character people love to hate. Previously best known to television audiences as the savvy assistant "Beverly" on "The Larry Sanders Show," Penny has appeared in feature films including "Absolute Power" and "What's Love Got to Do With It" and has been featured in television roles on "ER," Star Trek: Deep Space Nine," "Frasier," "The Practice," and many, many more. Look for Penny in ABC's new family drama series "October Road" in spring of 2007. In addition to her grandmother, Alzheimer's also claimed her mother-in-law.

Times You Don't Remember...
Times I Won't Forget
Christina Fuller

Eight years now and I can still remember with perfect clarity the moment I found out that my grandmother had been diagnosed with Alzheimer's Disease. I was in my sophomore year of college and my sister was in her senior year of high school. We knew she had not been feeling well and was having some memory problems, but nothing could have prepared me for the magnitude of this devastating disease.

"Girls," I remember my dad saying, "I went to the neurologist with your grandmother and he thinks she might have Alzheimer's Disease." I was surprised by the strength my dad showed that day. After all, this was his mother he was talking about. But he openly shared the details of her appointment, telling us that she couldn't remember her birth date or the current year. Yet when she was asked her grandchildren's names, she responded right away: "Christina and Joy."

When I heard this I smiled. My grandmother had always been the rock of my family, the ideal minister's wife. She exemplified love, kindness, and acceptance. She loved family and she raised her four children to stick close together. For a grandmother, no one could wish for better.

To say we were two peas in a pod would be putting it mildly. I was her first grandchild and her namesake. Every summer my parents would drop off my sister and me in Atlanta with my grandparents. But we spent most of our time with my grandmother. I was a charter member of her "clean plate club." To become a member, you had to eat all of your food. I loved to make her laugh, and my grandmother thought I was pretty funny, even if no one else thought so. When my grandfather would come home, she would repeat what I'd said, and he'd laugh, too. She was the first person who gave me confidence.

I remember with fondness the day she came to me and said, "You're 13 now, so today I will teach you the 23rd Psalm." She taught me, just as she had taught my aunt before me. We practiced for hours until I could recite the Psalm with poise and ease. Today, the 23rd Psalm remains etched in my memory, a reminder of a lovely moment when, in my grandmothers' eyes, I transitioned into womanhood.

Now that my grandmother was sick, what was going to happen to our family? What was going to happen to me? I had to hear my grandmother's voice when I called. She still had to meet me at the front door with a hug when I visited. I refused to eat anyone else's green beans! My life would never be the same, and I could not imagine that I would ever recover from this news.

I blamed my entire family for her illness. Why did she have to prepare breakfast and dinner? Why couldn't my grandfather iron his own shirts? I should have helped her clean up more. It was easier to blame a person than to blame an illness. While I played the blame game, my younger sister was more practical. "Is it hereditary?" she asked. But I only had one question, "When can I see grandma?"

When I saw her, two weeks after hearing of her diagnosis, I was shocked. She didn't look like a person who had Alzheimer's Disease; she looked and sounded the way she always had. She asked me about school. We talked about shopping together and when I was coming to Atlanta to visit. Obviously, the doctors didn't know what they were talking about, because my grandmother couldn't have Alzheimer's. She knew exactly who I was.

A few moments later, when she had difficulty remembering what day it was, the hard, cold truth slapped me in the face. Today she would remember that we loved to shop together and that I was in college, but after a few months, would she still remember?

The saving grace for my family was my dad's younger brother. While the rest of us were flailing in the wind, not knowing what to do about my grandmother's decline, he stepped forward, sacrificed his career and relocated to Georgia to live with my grandparents. His ideas about her care were radical. He believed that as long as my grandmother was around, we were going to give her the best possible care, and that care included a physical, mental and dietary regimen. He implemented his plan with passion and dedication. He lovingly nicknamed my grandmother "the soldier." She was at war and she had to fight for as long as she could.

Her first step was joining the Senior Center. My grandmother, who had never worn a pair of pants in her life, was riding the stationary bike, lifting weights, and taking a geriatric swim class. Although her memory was fading, it was as if she had a new lease on life. She also ate fresh vegetables and very little sugar and sodium. She balked at this, but soon she got used to it. I must admit that I secretly gave her an ice cream cone every now and then. She's always had a sweet tooth, and it was tough to go cold turkey! To keep her thinking, we would sit with her as she read the newspaper and wrote her name. In comparison to the exercise program and dietary restrictions, this was the most difficult for her. She didn't want to do it, but if I replaced a sales circular with the newspaper, she would agree to read. For awhile she even continued to travel with my grandfather.

As valiantly as we fought to keep her from deteriorating, it was inevitable. Eventually, the exercising and reading stopped. As she began to decline, we were forced to make some tough choices about her care. As a family we made a commitment that we would never send my grandmother to a nursing home. We are lucky to have found great nurses who are truly compatible with my grandmother. While it was a struggle in the beginning, now they seem to understand what she needs, even though she can't ask. It is wonderful that she can still be in the same home with my grandfather, her husband of 61 years. She doesn't talk much now, but whenever my grandfather walks into the room, she lights up and she calls his name. We still hold onto our healthy eating plan, and she still enjoys the occasional ice cream cone.

In spite of it all, we try to maintain the traditions and values that she taught us. We still celebrate Christmas as a family with her right there by our side, and even if she can't open her gifts and couldn't care less what we give her, it's our way of showing her that she continues to have meaning in our lives.

But with any serious illness, there are moments when all of the efforts at normalcy can't mask the truth, and sometimes this hits me hard. There are times when it takes everything I have to visit my grandmother, not because I don't love her, but because it is so hard to see her as she is today. She is a shell of the vibrant, strong, loving woman with the beautiful voice and smile that could light up a room.

In my mind, I can still hear her humming as she walked through the house and I can remember how beautiful she looked in her Sunday morning dress. I know that I can't get those moments back, but I don't want to. I would much rather look back on them with appreciation that for a moment, however brief, I was blessed to have her in my life.

I would have wanted her at my wedding, and to have been able to talk to the children I will have someday. For every special person who now enters my life, I am filled with sadness that they will never truly get to know my grandmother, but I can share her through my memories. They will last a lifetime. Even now, there are moments when my grandmother looks right into my eyes and calls me by name. It's those moments that matter most, and it lets me know that even though she has lost so many memories, inside she knows who I am and that the love we share will last forever.

Christina Fuller is a native of Greenville, South Carolina and a graduate of Brenau University. In addition to her work as marketing writer for a Greenville-based telecommunications company, she has contributed articles to the *Times Upstate* and *Greenville News* and has written for a national greeting card company. An avid reader and professionally trained singer, Fuller is preparing to write her first novel titled "*Praise the Mouth Almighty.*"

Grampa Forgets

Marcia Berneger

We always went to Chen's when we visited Grandma and Grandpa and we always started with its Won Ton soup. That's when it happened.

"Look what Grandpa's doing!" My little brother Bobby giggled and pointed across the table. We all stared as Grandpa ladled his soup … into his teacup. I giggled as well. I was only ten. I didn't realize yet.

My eyes circled the table: Mom was hushing Bobby; Dad stared into his own soup bowl and Grandma—her mouth was smiling, but her eyes—they were so sad. I didn't understand why, but what Grandpa did wasn't supposed to be funny. I stopped giggling and quietly finished my soup.

"Grandpa forgets things," was all Mom said.

We saw Grandma and Grandpa again just after my eleventh birthday. I was as tall as Grandpa now, even though I hadn't grown much. I wasn't sure, but I thought maybe he was shrinking. I didn't know people could do that. I raced up to Grandpa, but he just stared at me, his eyebrows wrinkling in confusion. Didn't he recognize me? After a long moment, he smiled. "Come give your Grandpa a hug, Stevie," he whispered. His blank stare haunted me for days.

Each visit brought more worrisome changes in Grandpa. Like the time he heated his coffee in the toaster oven instead of the microwave. What a mess; his mug melted all over the place! Or when he charged from the bathroom, clutching his toothbrush and a tube of shampoo. I tried not to giggle as he grumbled about the awful tasting toothpaste.

By the time I was twelve I knew something was terribly wrong. It was more than "Grandpa forgets things." Cornering my mom, I demanded the truth. My eyes locked onto hers. Tears pooled in her eyes and spilled down her anguished face. What had I done? Was Grandpa dying? But I had to know. Glancing away, I spoke softly, "Please Mom, what's wrong with Grandpa?"

"Grandpa has Alzheimer's," she whispered.

Alzheimer's? I'd heard about that. Old people get it and they forget stuff. But Grandpa sometimes forgets me!

"What will happen to Grandpa?" I asked.

"He will continue to forget."

"Until?"

"Until he can't remember where he is or what he's doing," she replied. "He won't always remember you, Stevie. Or even me." Sadness shrouded my mom. I hugged her. She squeezed me so hard I thought I would break in half.

"Can I help Grandpa remember us?"

Mom shook her head. "I don't think so. But right now he still knows us. We'll visit more often." I grew afraid. "Mom, what if I forget Grandpa?" Suddenly my own memories seemed fuzzy. Mom pulled out a big box from the closet. "Photographs are memories." I didn't understand. I ran my fingers through the pile of pictures in the box. Mom held one up.

"I remember this!" I said, grabbing the photo. There was Grandpa and me riding in the engine of the big steam train. He held me up while I blew the whistle.

"And this one!" reaching for another picture. "And this one!" Soon I had eight pictures laid out on the bed. There was Grandpa holding me for the very first time, Grandpa reading to me, and one of us just laughing together. Maybe these will help Grandpa remember, I thought. I dug deeply into the box and pulled out more memories. We found an empty photo album and I carefully placed each treasure onto a page. On our next visit, I scampered up into Grandpa's big brown chair and snuggled next to him.

"What do you have in your book, Robbie?" He smiled at me.

Gulping down the lump in my throat, I smiled back. Robbie was my uncle's name.

"It's a book of memories, Grandpa." I said, opening the album.

"I don't remember very well any more," he sighed.

I pointed to the first picture. "I'll help you, Grandpa."

Grandpa stared at that picture for a long time. A smile slowly spread across his face. "I remember that train whistle. It was sure loud, wasn't it, Stevie?"

Marcia Berneger is a second grade teacher by day and a wife, mother of two teenage sons and writer by night. She has been published in the *San Diego Union Tribune* and *Highlights Magazine* and has had a children's story and a poem included in two different literary anthologies.

Grandma's Love

Tamara Scully

It was her 90th birthday. She still smiled when I visited and she recognized Aaron, my son. But she was only Grandma in glimpses now. Alzheimer's Disease had robbed her of time and place and even person. Yet still, I wanted to share with her. I wanted her advice. So I talked and I asked, and she responded the best she was able. Her prized possession was an old afghan she made long ago. It was one of hundreds she created over her lifetime. She showed it to me again and again. A whole life filled with joy and pain, memories and remembrances, hopes and dreams was incorporated into this one gesture. It symbolized, I believe, all that she could no longer put into words.

Not so long ago, she was able to play hide-and-seek, to color and draw, and even to jump rope with her beloved great-grandchild, but now she could only smile at him and make simple statements. No more songs or jokes: communication consisted of "how big you are!" as she looked up—way up, for she was only four foot ten and Aaron was by then well on the way to being six feet tall. "Did you do your homework?" she asked him repeatedly. He answered in the affirmative, again and again. Her eyes sparkled just having him around. Even his photograph on a shelf in the room brought a big smile to her face.

As I reflected that day on all she had meant to me, I realized how she had enriched my life. This is not to say that she was perfect or that our intertwined lives had been without conflict. It was simply a statement of fact: she had shaped me, guided me, and influenced me greatly over the years.

I had a grandma when many others did not. My friends envied me. Their grandmas were far away, busy, "modern" women or, perhaps, deceased. Mine was present, and to us she was the "stereotypical grandma." Grandma baked and cooked our meals. She did laundry and planted flowers. She crocheted afghans and sweaters, sewed her own curtains. She belonged to several seniors' groups and enjoyed the company of family, friends and neighbors. She was a social person, playing cards and going to dinner weekly with her friends. She was active in the local senior citizens' clubs, donating hand-crafted items for fundraising events, baking cakes for meetings and driving other seniors to lunch.

Despite Alzheimer's Disease slowly taking her away, she still had her special friends. One other resident at the assisted living facility (that she now called "home") had formed a special attachment to my grandmother. Ruth and Grandma would hold hands, meet one another at meal times, and sit next to each other in the community room. As we accompanied Grandma to the dining room for lunch one afternoon, we stopped several doors down. Grandma was looking for Ruth. Not finding her, she rushed (even with her walker she was fast) to the dining area and right over to Ruth, who was already sitting at their assigned table. Gesturing for us to fol-low, she said "my friend," and "my daughter, my son" as a means of introducing us. Although we'd met Ruth many times previously and although Grandma hadn't quite been able to find the correct relationship terms to describe us, we knew the introduction was a heartfelt one.

Grandma was always there for me. Now, I realized, she was still there, incorporating her family as much as she could into her new world. Every visit we made now was just as important as the ones we had made regularly, before the disease forced so much to change. In fact, maybe the visits were more important, allowing Grandma to untangle enough of the web of her illness to briefly recollect the long and binding history we all shared.

Throughout the years, it never seemed to be a bad time to visit Grandma or to ask a favor. She was never too busy to attend to our needs. She always seemed happy to have us around. She was the one I would seek out when the world was cruel, when other kids were hurtful, or when I felt lonely. Just the atmosphere at her home could make the world right again for me. I still can hear the screen door banging shut, the chirping of the birds in the birdbath, the smell of pies baking, tomato sauce cooking and fragrant flowers blooming, mingled in the late afternoon air. Lemonade, ice cream, and cooling off in the sprinkler were simple pleasures not easily forgotten.

Now Grandma's life had changed. Her world was reduced to a bedroom to call her own and some common rooms to share with other patients. Grandma could no longer do all of those everyday things that made up my memories of our time together, but she was still taking care of us, even now, in many small ways.

During afternoon snack, Grandma seemed content as she was served her cookies and juice. But being Grandma, she flagged down the server and pointed to Aaron, and then to a cup, indicating that he, too, needed a snack. Once he had been served, she then smiled, nodded, and said "thank you." Then they both started eating. "Good," she said, clearly enjoying this snack she shared with her great-grandson, and watching closely to make sure that he was enjoying it as well.

Leaving Grandma that day, we made sure she was occupied and that the staff knew we were leaving. We kissed her goodbye, and I said "I love you." She puckered up to kiss me, and even grabbed Aaron for another. She insisted on walking to the door of the room as we walked down the hallway, waving goodbye until we were out of sight. She was still being a caretaker to her family even as she now needed care.

It wasn't until she was well into her 80s that Grandma began to slow down. It wasn't the slowing down that caused us concern. It was the subtle personality changes that seemed to insidiously invade her everyday activities. First, she began to close her draperies, not wanting "those nosy neighbors" to see her. Then, her friends began to "not want to sit with me and not call me." Next, her family began "to want me dead."

At first, we thought that the new neighbors might actually be nosy, and that her friends maybe did sit at a different table during the senior citizens' lunch. But when she began to verbally attack us, her family, we had our first clear clue that something was not right. Her angry outbursts, so unlike the woman we knew, became harsh. This woman, whose idea of profanity was to say "sugar," was now using words we didn't realize she even knew. And she started to walk away from family gatherings, accusing us of not really wanting her around. We knew then that something was very wrong.

After a complete medical and psychiatric evaluation, Grandma was diagnosed with Alzheimer's Disease and depression. A short-term stay in a psychiatric unit, where she was put on medications, seemed to help her distress. She was soon stable enough to leave the hospital, but we knew we could not let her return home, so we found her a place where they specialized in the care of those with dementia, a place that became a new home to her. She was comfortable, cared for, and had plenty of social contact. We tried to make her room a reminder of the home she had maintained for so many years. Photographs of all the great-grandchildren, her familiar hairbrush and comb, her favorite rocking chair and stool and the old afghan she always used to cover her legs at night were all part of our attempt to bring to her a sense of familiarity.

Just after her 90th birthday, Grandma began to suffer from increasingly serious medical issues. Fluctuating blood pressure led to falls. Internal bleeding, mysterious but steady, necessitated blood transfusions every three months. Her mind became increasingly befuddled and agitation began to override any daily joy. Grandma was entering the end-stages of Alzheimer's Disease, and we addressed the decisions regarding the end of her life.

As we moved Grandma to the last home she would ever know, a skilled nursing facility, we decided to withhold treatment for the chronic health conditions that could cause her death before Alzheimer's Disease inevitably would. We declined the use of feeding tubes were they to become necessary. We did consent to an IV for fluids, once, but not the second time.

At this point, she no longer looked comfortable. She was always pulling, picking, and tugging. Grabbing at anyone or anything, she could no longer work her once-nimble hands. As the disease had ravaged her mind, it was now visibly ravaging her body. She lost the ability to swallow all but the softest foods, pureed to prevent choking. She became thin and frail and unable to walk. She spent her days in a reclining chair, locked in to prevent falls.

The reversal of our roles as she became dependent and we became her guardians revealed to us the finite nature of this lifetime, and in doing so, it enriched our own lives. We became more aware of the passage of time, of the connectedness we all share and of the grace of the present moment. No longer was Grandma the source of comfort to us. We tried to comfort her as best we could. She no longer had any means of imparting her wisdom to us. We, instead, tried to use what she had taught us to bring her peace in her final days.

For her 91st birthday, we did not speak of birthday cake or parties. Instead, we brought everyone in the family to see her for what we all knew would be the last gathering. This time she managed a smile but not much else, sleeping most of the time we were there. It was a difficult visit for all of us. We later talked about how

Grandma no longer could do all the things we associated with her and how it was time for her to leave this life and pass on to the next.

Mercifully, her death was not far off. We wanted her to be released from the body and mind which no longer served her and we wanted to be free to remember the Grandma she was, not agonize over decisions for the body she no longer seemed to inhabit. My grieving for her had begun long before her actual death. Over the several long years of watching the disease take her, I had said my good-byes many times and I had made peace with the decisions, choices, and mistakes that we had made along the way.

Using the wisdom, insight, and kindness that Grandma had taught us through all the years we shared, we gave her what we thought was the best care we could. That, I think, was the ultimate legacy. We attempted to give back to her just a portion of the love she had given to us. And I think, somehow, she knew.

Grandma died on the day that I bought my house; the precise time of death was the minute the sellers put the keys in my hands. That, I choose to believe, was her parting gift to me. Seeing me safely home, she went home. We buried Grandma with her handmade, beloved afghan, the last object she was able to recognize. It brought us great comfort to "tuck her in" one final time.

Tamara Jean Scully is a farmer, local foods advocate and freelance writer. A 1988 graduate of Wake Forest University, she lives in northwestern New Jersey with her husband, son and cats. Her articles have appeared in *Skylands Visitor Magazine, Organic Producer Magazine* and many other publications.

The Alzheimer's Journey

Dawn Eason

On December 2, 1997 my beloved grandfather passed away. His dying words to his three daughters were, "Take care of your Mama." He knew something we didn't: that grandmother was suffering from Alzheimer's Disease.

I can't say he hadn't tried to talk to us about it. He would make comments about how she just couldn't remember anything or about the things she was doing which were so out of character. We were deeply in denial and found ourselves getting angry with him for making such accusations against an aging woman who simply might not be as sharp as she once was.

I can't say we hadn't at least suspected something was wrong with her. We noticed that the things she worked so hard for all her life suddenly didn't hold much interest for her and simple tasks were now harder for her to complete. For instance, Ma Ma had always been a meticulous housekeeper. We started seeing dust building up and carpets that had not been vacuumed. We chalked it up to her not feeling well; we jumped in and started cleaning her house. We also noticed how she had stopped sewing, one of her favorite pastimes. We tried to convince ourselves that she was just tired, and maybe physically a little under the weather. It wasn't until my grandfather's death that we realized exactly what we were dealing with, and what he had been dealing with.

Alzheimer's Disease is the saddest condition I have ever encountered. To watch the person you have known and loved your entire life slowly slip away is heartbreaking. The saddest part is that even though she is gone, she is still here. You are left with only a shell of the person who was such a vital part of your life.

We soon realized that someone needed to stay with Ma Ma on a 24-hour basis. She had started wandering, and we knew it wasn't safe to leave her alone. Each of her three daughters rotated shifts every day for four years. She became progressively worse over this time, and her personality changed. What once had been the most loving woman in the world was becoming a stranger to us, often aggressive, with mood swings nothing like we had ever witnessed from her. We had to keep telling ourselves that her actions and words were not from her but from the disease that was robbing her of her memory. Finally, it became evident that she would need to be placed in a full time care facility.

Please, please, please, don't ever let anyone make you feel guilty for placing your loved one in a skilled facility. It is a tough decision to make, probably one of the toughest you will ever make in your life. But you have to understand that it's okay to offer your loved one the care she needs. More importantly, don't let others who have not walked in your shoes judge you for the decisions you make. There's no doubt that other people condemned my family for its decision to place Ma Ma in a care facility, but until you actually live through an ordeal such as this, you have no clue what you would do.

If the time does come to move your loved one, find a facility that specializes in Alzheimer's care. As with most Alzheimer's patients, my grandmother needed to be in a locked facility and her physical health was still very good for someone in her 70's, so she needed different care from what was offered in a traditional nursing home setting. We were fortunate enough to find a wonderful facility in a nearby town.

After 3½ years in this special facility, my grandmother's condition progressed to a point where she no longer needed Alzheimer's care. The family was told that she would have to be moved. She was placed in a regular nursing home facility here in town. What we thought would be a positive change quickly turned in another direction. If you have had any dealings with advanced Alzheimer's, you know that the patient can lose some physical functions, one of which may be the ability to swallow. On her second day in the new facility, we were told that the aides were afraid to feed my grandmother due to her choking so easily, and that they would not put in a feeding tube because her living will directed that such treatment be withheld. We had always said that we would not put her through that, but when it came down to the wire, we couldn't let her starve to death. We were somewhat relieved that Ma Ma had made that decision for herself, years earlier. Our only option was to go to the nursing home and feed her.

Over the course of the next three months, Ma Ma lost more than thirty pounds. She was always a petite woman and her weight loss caused her to fall below one hundred pounds. While this was a trying time for the family, we were fortunate that we got to spend a lot of time with her. I've read enough about Alzheimer's to know that the patient eventually gets to the point of being unable to recognize family and friends, but I believe that Ma Ma knew us when we came in the room. I remember going to feed her at lunch one day after her condition had worsened. She hadn't uttered a sound in days, but when I walked into the room, she opened her eyes, looked up at me and said, "Hey, sugar!" When I would ask her if she loved me, she told me she did. She would relax when we were in the room with her, and she would even open her eyes to look around occasionally, as if she were checking so see if we were still there. I could see in her eyes that there was some sort of recognition, and nothing can make me believe otherwise. Keep talking to your loved one just as you always have. You never know how she'll respond, and those precious few words my grandmother spoke will forever live in my heart.

Alzheimer's Disease tests your faith in God. I was raised by a loving, Christian family and went to church with my grandparents when I was a young girl. I grew up in the church but over the years I drifted away. I could tell it bothered my grandmother and I know that she sent many prayers to Heaven on my behalf. I still had the values and beliefs that I had grown up with, but I couldn't help asking God why this woman, who had been so faithful to Him and lived the best Christian life she possibly could, ended up with such a hopeless disease. I was bitter at times because of it.

In 2001, at the insistence of my daughter, then four years old, we started attending church—the same church I grew up in, where my grandparents had been longtime members. I quickly realized how much I had been missing and how spiritually dead I had become. We started attending regularly and have recently joined the church. I have come to realize that God has a plan for everything and everyone and it's not necessary for us to understand. I know that he used Ma Ma for a greater purpose and we may never know exactly what that purpose was. I sometimes wonder if it was to get her family back into the church she loved so much. You see, we've all started attending church each week, and we have a much closer relationship with God. Although she never told me, I know that was one of those many prayers my grandmother sent to Heaven. Whatever His reason, I know she was more than willing to let Him work through her.

God was present throughout her illness. We had asked that my grandmother be moved to a local hospice facility. We got the call on Thanksgiving Day that a bed was available there for her. We were told that two other people were in need of the same bed, but for whatever reason they chose her. We didn't realize that there was a two week maximum stay at the facility and we were even told that based on her condition, she would more than likely be moved back to the nursing home. We put our trust in God that things were working out and He was getting ready to end her suffering.

Eleven days after moving to the hospice and eight years to the day that we buried my grandfather, my beloved grandmother passed away. For all the years of suffering she had endured, God took her from this world in the most peaceful manner possible; she was surrounded by her family. It was a beautiful ending to her story and I'm so thankful for the opportunity to have been by her side.

If you find that you have a loved one facing Alzheimer's Disease, you will inevitably learn a lot about yourself. You will learn to have patience, endurance and strength. Your faith will be tested and hopefully, strengthened. Alzheimer's Disease is sadly a death sentence for the person diagnosed, so make the most of the precious time that remains. Say and do the things you need to before it's too late. Do whatever it takes to guarantee peace for yourself after it's all over.

Dawn Eason is a mother of two who works for a construction company in North Carolina. This story was created as part of the author's own healing process in dealing with her grandmother's passing.

Firehouse

Claire Carpenter

I do not claim to know my grandfather, Robert Lesley Stephenson, even well enough to do him the credit his life deserves. But I know that Papa is surprised to still be alive, the only one out of his four brothers, still confident that he should have died six years ago. "No Stephenson man lives past the age of eighty-three," was one of his one liners when he was eighty-two. He is now an eighty-nine year old great-grandfather in a nursing home, and although no longer strong of body, he is still the same witty man who saves his one-liners for the right moment. He is Les, and he is my Papa.

For example, a week before my grandparents moved from the assisted living facility to the nursing home, Papa overheard my mother telling his wife, "We're going to try to keep you together. That's the most important thing." He suddenly perked up and turned to my father and said, "Are they talking about burial plots?" His eyes twinkled in a way that only happens with grandfathers. My father laughed, not sure why he was surprised at my grandfather's wit. After all, he still recognizes and loves his family and is still happy wherever his wife is.

Long before my grandfather's Alzheimer's diagnosis, he had planned to take my grandmother, my mother and me on a trip to France as my graduation present. The four of us would spend two weeks making a circuit of the country. Although the diagnosis wouldn't come until after the trip, my grandparents had already noticed Papa's growing uncertainty and wanted to pull out. They knew what burdens older people could be and had always tried to be sensitive to that, even when they were seventy and still so young, but my mother and I convinced them to come anyway. It would be fine. They couldn't miss going overseas for what could be the last time.

The trip should have gone easily enough. My grandparents were experienced travelers. Ever since their retirement, they had spent three months every other year traveling through Europe, snapping photographs of major landmarks and staying in good hotels. Our hotel in Paris was a converted section of an apartment building with a lovely atrium in the center, and a small foyer served as the breakfast patio. It felt right from the moment we stepped in. My grandparents napped on a king-sized bed while my mother and I wandered the streets around our block to fight our jetlag. Over the next two days my mother and I hurried to all the major tourist sites and smaller museums. We regretted leaving my grandparents behind in the hotel room or in a café, but they seemed content. They had seen it all before several times.

Our third night in Paris, I was asleep when my grandfather walked out of the hotel. I didn't know anything had happened until the next morning when my mother looked exceptionally ragged and my grandmother was frazzled with a headache. Papa, too, I remember, was agitated. He was usually such a calm man. I knew something was wrong.

He had evidently woken from a particularly vivid dream, convinced that a little boy was trapped in a fire upstairs. He needed to get to a firehouse immediately, so he padded barefoot out through the breakfast atrium to the front door. My mother somehow woke up, instinctively glanced toward her parents' bed and found the right side was empty. Five frantic minutes later, she found him down the street, asking a Frenchman for directions to the nearest firehouse. As she ushered Papa back to our room, he insisted he hadn't been dreaming and that we needed to help the boy. "There's a fire, right now!" he repeated, over and over, even the morning after. My mother eventually decided to participate in his reality, just to calm him down and said, "We called the right people, and they helped the little boy. Everything is fine now."

That was almost five years ago, when his dreams started to become reality. His traveler's mind, once composed of detailed itineraries and calculations of mileage, was now breaking down into a jumble of places and people who only existed in dreams. I remember being afraid that I was losing my grandfather, that he was becoming something new and different.

The early stages of Alzheimer's can do that; can create the illusion that a person is changing, regressing, losing himself in a muddle of thoughts. My grandfather's muddle happened to be dreams he described so well that I wanted to believe they were real. He tried to be patient with us while we explained why and how his dreams weren't real. He spent hours mulling things over in his head, and it was when I saw him carefully outlining his reasons for his perceived reality that I knew he hadn't changed. He was still methodical and accounted for every detail that his mind could discern, trying to make a case for his own reality.

The last time I saw my grandfather, he was lying flat on his back in the nursing home. His twin bed had been pushed up against my grandmother's so that the two formed a sort of oversized queen. He looked uncomfortably stiff but not unhappy. He was calm, no longer the grandfather from the trip to France who tended toward belligerence and who yearned to be believed.

His eyes looked gentle through the same thick bifocals he wore in my baby pictures. The thin wisps of his white hair lay smoothly across the top of his head. Papa smiled when he noticed me and my husband standing at the foot of his bed. I stepped forward and grasped his veined hand, and his squeeze was amazingly strong for an eighty-nine year old man.

"Mother has sent us to get you out of bed and into the dining room," I said into his ear. "I've heard from the aides that you can get yourself out of bed and into the wheelchair now, but do you want a little help this time?"

He smiled with appreciation but said no.

After several minutes, my own impatience prodded me to offer my help again as he had only shifted closer to the edge of the bed, but again he shook his head. With a sigh he said, almost absently, "I need to install one of those triangular handles above the bed. I think I could move a lot faster with one of those."

Only a year ago, he would have gone to his garage workshop and retrieved his electric drill and a few screws and set to work installing a handle. The finished work would be immaculate and impossible to remove without destroying the ceiling.

"Are you sure you don't need any help? We're perfectly willing," I said, sliding my arm under his shoulder.

"No, no." He closed his eyes and summoned energy for the next move. I'd never seen him do this and wished he would just open his eyes and do something normal. And he did. He looked right at me and said, "You'll have to yell 'fire' if you want me to move any faster than this," smiling the same as always.

And so ten minutes later, when little progress had been made, I said, "Papa, I'm sorry to say this, but there's a fire in here and we have to go now." He only smiled again and nodded, pretending he hadn't understood what I'd said. I wished I could just pick him up and place him in the wheelchair in one graceful movement. He has always been slow and methodical in everything though, and I couldn't and wouldn't want to change him now. I used to wonder if there was some unseen value in his slow ways; now I'm inclined to believe there was. Maybe he knew even before then that slow and steady wins the race.

He was still going slow and steady and about twenty minutes later, with the help of an aide, my husband, and my father, we got Papa into the wheelchair and pushed him down the hall to the dining room where his wife and daughter waited for him. As he leaned forward and kissed his wife on the cheek and squeezed her hand, I couldn't tell that he had Alzheimer's. In fact, if I hadn't known already, I would never have known. He was simply an old man who had grown frail of body but not of spirit. He was still aware of us, of life.

Later, he asked my father, "How much is this place costing me a month?" My father explained the price and that they had moved him from his house a few months ago, a look of satisfaction appeared on my grandfather's face.

"Is that so? That's good to know." He wasn't unhappy or confused but content because he had all that he needed right there in that very room.

The author is a Masters in Fine Arts candidate at Oregon State University and has received two awards for her nonfiction writing. Her fiction and nonfiction have appeared in *Miranda Literary Magazine, Four Hundred Words,* and *Lily Literary Review.*

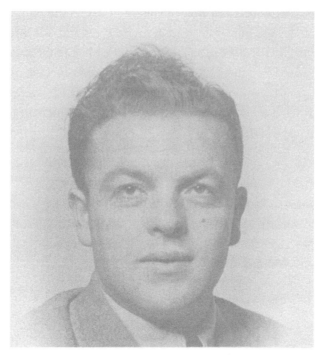

Leopold Van Dyke, page 91

Part IV
THE CAREGIVERS

What do we live for if not to make life less difficult for each other?

—*George Eliot*

Finding Comfort,
Strength and Inspiration
Francine Siegel

People often ask me why I chose to work with as difficult a population as Alzheimer's caregivers. The fact is I don't find it difficult, I find it rewarding and inspiring. I work with individuals, families, and groups in a way few people can: by sharing others' lives. As I share their care giving challenges and watch their powerful transformations, I find my own strength and I am inspired to continue the work.

I meet with family caregivers—spouses and adult children—in counseling sessions and support groups. It's hard for people to seek outside help, attend a support group with strangers or share the feelings that this disease brings on. Often, people don't come back after the first visit. When they do start coming regularly, sometimes months or even years after their first visit, they find they can carry on because of the comfort and support they receive. Some attend a support group for many years, watching the patient decline but also seeing their own strength grow. It is amazing that people are able to handle the toughest roles; it takes courage. Here are a few.

Stella, 75, is small and thin. Stella did not speak at all the first time she came to the support group. She cried gently throughout the session. She listened as Mary discussed her husband's repetitive questioning, as Anna discussed the many physical problems her husband was facing and her own back pain from lifting and moving him, and as Lenore discussed her husband's arguments with others in his nursing home. Stella cried. Each time she was asked to tell her story, she said she couldn't talk. She was an emotional wreck and did not know how she could go on. At the end of the 90 minute session, Stella stood up, slowly gathering wads of crumpled tissues. My group members encircled her, hugging and nodding and supporting her. I couldn't see her through the circle of loving arms. We had no idea of the stage, diagnosis, or condition of her family member. We didn't know anything about her life. All we knew was that she had to care for someone with dementia and could not find the strength to do so. I watched as she found comfort from the group after just one session.

Ruth, a big 88 year old woman, came regularly to group over many months. She dressed in unstylish clothing and carried a tote bag with notepads and markers. She was looking for answers to solve her problems. Ruth was tough, and you could see the anger in her eyes and face. She said, "No one, not anyone in group or outside can understand my pain." After all, she had had to care for her own parents as they aged, and her husband's mother, and was now caring for her husband as he slowly and progressively declined. Ruth resented her role. She was angry that her grown children and their grown children were not there for her, as she had always been for her own family. She even babysat for her great-grandson in her own home, two mornings a week. She told the group, "Sure, my kids have their own fine lives that *we struggled to give them*; they really don't care about me. No one does." She felt angry, weary and lonely.

There comes a time when the burden becomes too much for a caregiver and she needs to relinquish some of the chore to others. If Ruth's family wouldn't help her, there were social services and skilled nursing facilities that would take over. I hoped the group members would convince Ruth that she was doing too much. They know what it is to care for a sick patient; they know what it is to "lose" a husband who is still there; they know how it hurts. But, because of her stoic resistance, group members weren't really fond of Ruth. So when she did not show up for two meetings, I encouraged the members to call her. They found out Ruth had suffered a heart attack. The telephone calls from group members caused a change in Ruth. She felt caring from the group, began to accept outside help and looked for ways to maintain her new strength.

Ann is a shy woman of 63 caring for her 85 year old father. Ann looked like the oldest in the group even though she was the youngest. She had lived all her life alone with her parents in a small, shabby home. Her father was an angry, abusive man when he was well. Now Alzheimer's Disease made him angrier and more demanding. He no longer made sense when he spoke. He could no longer walk. The hospital bed and boxes of care items were squeezed into their living room. Ann continued to care for him, staying by his side, liquefying his food, feeding him with a tube and lifting him with a huge contraption. When Ann told her story the others in group squirmed. He needed nursing home care. Ann would not think of it. We watched her age and lose weight. We watched her dedicate her life to a father who was cruel to her.

As Ann's father declined, we saw a miraculous turnaround. Ann came to realize that she was capable and strong. She could manage her household, hire health care aides, deal with nurses, doctors, accountants, lawyers. She told the group about her successes, about entitlements she located and ways to speak up for her needs. Others learned from her. Ann learned that she could have left her home and taken care of herself years ago. Now she began to explore: buying new clothing, learning to use a computer, doing volunteer work, joining a singles golf club. With therapy and the support group, Ann was able to speak her thoughts and feelings. She was able to face her new life and let in people and joy. I watched Ann mature and I felt stronger with her.

I wish there was a magic pill for my clients that would make their lives better. I don't have immediate solutions. I ask them to talk about what it feels like to be a caregiver. Together, we examine what people can control and what they can't. We look at what works and what doesn't work, as each person tells his or her own story. I see the enormous courage of caregivers. The members are comforted by this courage and learn that they can grow strong. It is a powerful lesson. The amazing transformations I see in their lives helps explain the inspiration I get from my work. I am grateful for the opportunity to work with these "difficult" people.

Francine is a Licensed Clinical Social Worker and psychotherapist in private practice on Long Island, New York. After a career in publishing, she earned a Master's Degree in Social Work and continues with postgraduate training in Family Therapy, Group Therapy and Eldercare. Her work includes leading caregiver support groups and bereavement and discussion groups for seniors.

Breaking up with My Gardenia
Valerie M. Smith

Grief associated with a death may be overwhelming in the beginning, and gradually lessen. Grief associated with a chronic illness seems to go on and on. Your feelings may shift back and forth between hope that the person will get better and anger and sadness over an irreversible condition.

—The 36-Hour Day: A Family Guide to
Caring for Persons with Alzheimer's Disease

One of my best friends, who adopted a child and then within nine months gave birth, "brokeup" with her cat of five years when the demands of parenting and working full time *and* being a pet owner became too great. She still fed him and brought him to the vet and took care of him in every way he needed; she just decided he could no longer be a central figure in her emotional life. Umbro didn't seem to take umbrage at his new status. It was a successfully completed, if somewhat painful, breakup.

I recently had a similar, although decidedly less successful, breakup experience.

Last year my household consisted of my husband and I, an elderly cat, fifteen goldfish, an assortment of what I call "easy care" houseplants and an eclectic mix of antique and Ikea furniture.

This year, my home has expanded to include my two elderly and fragile parents, their two cats (one formerly feral and still skittish, one a large and wandering Manx), three thousand African Violets, a few Christmas Cacti, a lopsided *Sanseviera laurentii* and fifteen tons of well-worn furniture. Our three bedroom, one and one-half bath home now fits like a size five shoe on a size eight foot.

I could go into detail about learning how to live with my father's blindness: anticipating what he might not see but will probably need to find, ensuring nothing is moved from its usual position in the house so that it does not become a hazard; remembering to put the orange juice and the butter dish back into the exact same place in the fridge so he can find them when he wants them; reading mail aloud, finding phone numbers, remembering to leave an extra roll of toilet paper available so that if it runs out when I'm not home he won't be fumbling around in a potentially messy situation. But I won't go into those details. I could also go into details about the precarious nature of his heart condition, his increasingly wobbly walk, his most recent dangerous bout of bronchitis, but what would be the point?

I could tell about learning to live with my mother's memory loss: the strategies I have taught myself to better respond to her some-times-mercurial needs; the difficult dynamics that arise as the care-giver becomes the cared-for. But I won't go into those details either. Not now, because they are still too close to the heart. Instead, I will tell you the story of breaking up with my gardenia.

Sometimes it is helpful to find other outlets for your frustrations: talking to someone, cleaning closets, or chopping wood—whatever ways you have used in the past to cope with your frustrations. A vigorous exercise program, a long walk, or taking a few minutes to relax totally may be help to you.

—The 36-Hour Day: A Family Guide to Caring for Persons with Alzheimer's Disease

It all began sometime last spring when I impulsively bought a shiny, dark green gardenia. Once a year, usually in late winter or early spring, gardenias produce waxy, snow-white blooms that fill the air with the heady aroma of a summer garden. To smell one is to be transported back to the heat of youthful summers. The plant beckoned me from among rows of healthy greenery in our local nursery. The greenhouse was redolent with heat and moisture and the clean scent of potting soil. I admit that I was somewhat overcome.

The gardenia resided in the house until the weather warmed and all houseplants that could safely be removed were transported to their summer home on an old picnic table under the large maple tree in the back yard. Although grass would not grow under the maple, houseplants seemed to thrive in its shade. The gardenia and all the other houseplants flourished in their summer arbor, as did the interior of the house, with its luxury of additional space. Come fall, as the days grew shorter and summer warmth melted into cooler autumn nights, the houseplants came back in. With their return, the house was once again overflowing, and my care giving expanded to meet their needs as well.

I suppose I was just overwhelmed the day I walked into the dining room and noticed the now pitiful state of the once glowing gardenia. Its leaves were yellowed; others had fallen off and littered the dining room floor. I touched the plant's droughty soil. That's when it struck me. Instead of continuing to care haphazardly for the plant, I could, like my friend with her cat, simply end the situation. I grabbed the heavy pot and marched straight outside to the compost bin. I confess I would never have contemplated such a drastic act without the reassuring graveyard of the compost pile, knowing that what little life the gardenia had left would be sacrificed for a noble cause: feeding next year's tomatoes and beans. Without a moment's hesitation and with a feeling of great relief, I tipped the plant out of its pot and into the bin. "I'm breaking up with you," I said over my shoulder as I tramped back to the house through a carpet of moldering autumn leaves.

Several hours later I saw the gardenia, repotted and trimmed, sitting defiantly in the middle of the back yard. Curious, I asked my husband if he knew anything about it. "Well," he said with a broad smile, "I found the gardenia in the compost pile, and your mother and I repotted it and brought it back to life." His grin widened. How could I tell him I'd broken up with the gardenia and did not, under any circumstances, plan on resuscitating the relationship? "I can't take care of another thing right now," I said. "Something has to go, and unless you want to volunteer then I think it's the gardenia."

Several days later, my husband cheerfully announced that he had taken the gardenia to a friend's house for safe-keeping, confident that I would eventually claim it back. "She'll look after it, until you're ready to take it back," he assured me. I shrugged and shook my head and walked away in disbelief. The breakup was not going well.

Weeks later, the gardenia appeared on a friend's desk at work. "Look, I've got your gardenia," Betsy said, smiling broadly and gesturing like a magician's assistant toward the now glowing plant.

"Um, I see. Tony told me he'd taken it to your house."

"And I told him I'd take care of it, but now that it looks so great again, I thought you'd want it back." I tried to smile as I backed out of the room, keeping one eye firmly on the gardenia.

The very next morning I opened my office door to find the gardenia sitting squarely amidst the stacks of books and papers on my messy desk. Attached to it was a little yellow post-it note: "Remember Me? I'm back."

> A dementing illness does not suddenly end a person's
> capacity to experience love or joy, nor does it end her
> ability to laugh. And, although your life may often seem

filled with fatigue, frustration, or grief, your capacity for happier emotions is not gone either. Happiness may seem out of place in the face of trouble, but in fact it crops up unexpectedly.

—The 36-Hour Day: A Family Guide to
Caring for Persons with Alzheimer's Disease

I've never been good at breaking up. Most of my successful break-ups have required moves between states or across continents or oceans. Perhaps that was my mistake here. The gardenia sits calmly on the windowsill in my office. I water it twice weekly and it seems to be thriving. For now, we have declared a truce; it retains its leaves and I retain whatever good grace I can.

Valerie teaches English at Quinnipiac University. She enjoys reading, writing, gardening and is currently attempting to learn to play the piano.

Goodness Knows

Ruth Jones

I fell in love with him at my job. My affection for him grew over the year and a half we worked together. At first I admired his cute face. Blue eyes sparkled and danced around a short squat nose, two pale pink lines arcing slightly at the corners hinted at a smile and a sense of humor, and his expression was friendly and accepting. Short gray hair gelled and combed into neat rows, a respectable style for a former English teacher, was complemented by a preppy collared shirt and pleated pants. His voice, a rich bell-like tenor, rang out Boston roots. Bob and I seemed to have an instant rapport.

"Would you like to take a walk with me?" I asked.

He shrugged his shoulders, holding his hands up as if surprised by the question and surprised at his good fortune. "With such a pretty girl? Of course."

I began to look forward to seeing Bob. I often started my day at work in the large rotunda, florescent lights blaring over an enormous circular desk. The flurry of activity, ringing phones, rushing workers and blinking lights burdened my state of mind, anticipating a heavy workload ahead. I would spy Bob sitting calm and collected. I'd wave and smile. He would return my gesture by raising his eyebrows and forming his mouth into a capital "O." For a moment, my cloud of doom would evaporate.

Bob and I often didn't need words to express the fond esteem in which we held one another. When we looked into each other's eyes, we encountered all that was kind and good within. But there was also another reason why words were not used. Bob had Alzheimer's Disease. I met Bob, a resident, while working as a physical therapist at a nursing home.

Alzheimer's launches its victims on a steady journey of reverse development, its final destination, helplessness. Plaques form on the brain, short-circuiting its wiring. The process is gradual, robbing function like a crooked cashier stealing pennies and dimes from the cash drawer. At first, the losses are barely noticeable. Over time, they add up. In the early stages, victims are often able to hide their deficits. When evaluating a new patient, I must determine their mental status. There are abrupt, pointed questions, the intent of which is difficult to disguise: What is the date today? Can you tell me the name of this place? What year is it? Who is the president?

When I asked Bob who was the President, he replied with widening eyes, "Well that guy... I don't even want to think about him."

Our therapy sessions were enjoyable. Bob would begin by greeting me like an old friend. "Well there she is," he'd say, smiling, recognizing my face but not really knowing who I was. He complied with my requests for him to ride on the exercise bike, walk down the hallway or do some balance exercises on the parallel bars, no matter how strange they may have seemed to him.

"You want me to get on this thing... Walk down here... Okay, anything you say."

Bob often told jokes that made no sense. It didn't matter to me. The cluck of his chuckle, the shine of his blue eyes, his charming facial expressions were reward enough. I rarely saw him angry or frustrated. Bob's son visited frequently, bringing him favorite treats. "Pie? Oh, let's go have some pie right now," Bob would say, looking like a kid hearing the music of an ice cream truck. I wasn't surprised to learn from Bob's son that in addition to teaching, Bob worked with underprivileged and wayward youths after school. How can a disease that wreaks havoc with the human brain leave some aspects of character untouched? With Bob, I like to believe God would not allow the disease to take what was essentially *him*.

Bob negotiated with panache what I call the revolving door of healthcare: hospital to nursing home, back to hospital, to the nursing home again, but each time arriving back just a little bit sicker and a little more confused. When Bob fell and broke a hip, he could no longer walk and was confined to a wheelchair. I would stop and visit with him many mornings. He would take my hand in his and smile. His words no longer made sense but his touch satisfied. Once I saw an aide hand Bob a nutritional supplement in a paper carton. When the aide left, Bob offered his drink to the lady next to him.

The last time I saw him, he had arrived very lethargic from a visit to the hospital. I entered the patient dining room where the speech pathologist was trying to get Bob to eat. He sat in his wheelchair, head resting on the table, a tray of food untouched just beyond the top of his head.

"I can't get him to eat. He's really gone downhill this time." She shook her head. "Bob, wake up." No response. The other speech pathologist in the room looked over at us, her mouth forming a grim line.

"Bob!" I raised my voice like a schoolteacher trying to get the class's attention. "You have three beautiful women here wanting to talk to you."

Bob raised his head and opened his eyes to reveal the two blue gems they contained, and smiled wide. We all laughed. Then Bob put his head back down on the table. He died two days later.

In the world of medicine, nerve fibers malfunction, hips break, hearts stop beating, but the spirit remains untouched. The memory of that spirit in Bob still warms me today. I am happier and more comfortable walking this earth knowing that Bob walked it before me.

The author is a graduate of Northwestern University's School of Physical Therapy. She enjoys working with the geriatric population and is currently in practice at John Knox Village Retirement Community in Tampa, Florida. Ruth studied writing at the University of South Florida.

They Wanted Me to Tell You

Deborah Attix

In the 11 years I have worked as a clinical neuropsychologist at Duke University Medical Center, my patients with Alzheimer's Disease have taught me in their own unique, distinct ways how they best cope with the memory loss and functional limitations caused by the disease and how they wish to be treated by others. I pass along that information now to help provide insight and understanding to family members and friends who love someone struggling with Alzheimer's or dementia. I hope that you will consider this information and pass it on, too.

In my work I specialize in assessing the condition of patients with memory disorders and offer therapeutic intervention when appropriate. Neurologists, psychiatrists and general medicine physicians refer patients to me for comprehensive testing of memory and thinking skills, for assistance in differential diagnosis (i.e., is this Alzheimer's Disease, stroke, or depression), and for information about clinical course (e.g., is the patient getting worse or staying stable). Through my clinical intervention service, I teach patients how to compensate for memory problems and provide therapy to help them cope when their thought processes become impaired.

Through the intervention service, patients allow me to accompany them on a portion of their journey. For some, it is early in the course of their illness, at diagnosis and the first hints of memory loss. Others come to see me later, when mounting cognitive problems lead to less and less of an ability to function day to day and frustration and grief abound. In all cases, patients who come to see me have at least some awareness of their losses and they are struggling to deal with the changes they are experiencing.

Fatigue and grief color the landscape of dementia for many patients and even more caregivers. Patients who retain insight see how their loved ones struggle with the *disease*, but often interpret this as their loved ones' struggle with *them*. They perceive themselves as a burden; too often their sense of self-worth is tied up with their diminishing capacities. And yet the person, *the self*, still exists despite declining cognition, and can even thrive despite progressive intellectual loss, if there is careful attention paid to validation of the *person*. Fatigue, grief, sadness, anger and despair, even resentment and futility all make appearances in the dementia journey. But the *person* will more fully thrive if they know, or sense, that while the illness authors these feelings, *they* do not.

Despite the pain of loss, in the end most wives, husbands, daughters, sons, sisters, brothers, and other caregivers would never give up their time with the patient suffering from dementia. They manage to see their loved ones, not just the disease. As a therapist, being present on part of the journey is an immense privilege.

Over time, my groups and individual patients have become more vocal about what they want me to convey when I give talks or write about this disease. Here are some of their thoughts, ideas, and beliefs:

- We know there are things we cannot do. It is important to focus on what we can do, so that we can continue to move forward.

- We do not like to be treated as if we were not there. Help people to interact with us appropriately.

- We feel safe when we are understood—when we are with other people who have similar problems or with people who understand that we can't always get the words out or stay on track. Sometimes it is like trying to see or hear through thick mosquito netting, other times it is clearer. It is not always the same and this is because of the illness, not because of how hard we try.

- We are here. Our memories and words might not always be, but we are.

Be sure to remember that people with dementia are not children. Their processing skills may be impaired, including their judgment skills. However, they have a lifetime of experience. While they may need significant guidance, direction and assistance, speak and interact with them in a way that allows them to retain as much dignity as possible.

Much to our delight, we have come to understand that patients with mild to moderate dementia are able to learn and benefit from specific therapeutic activities. It is fascinating to watch. Often, patients have a hard time recalling or relating the content of group therapy sessions even ten minutes after they end. Yet, after a short time, they can clearly relate major themes, their perception of benefit, and the specific content from group. Learning and benefit occur despite the memory deficit.

Patients with dementia are more than their memory. Indeed, information processing skills are not the same, function is not the same. But they are more than these things. They are still before you, being and feeling. Despair will happen. Work to recapture the joy and spirit that carries us through.

They wanted me to tell you. Pass it on.

Deborah Attix, Ph.D., ABPP/ABCN is the Director of the Duke Clinical Neuropsychology Service and the editor of the periodical *Geriatric Neuropsychology: Assessment and Intervention.*

Is My Mother Still Alive?

Judith Terzi

—

"Is my mother still alive?" my mother asked, as she frantically switched her hearing aid from one ear to the other, forgetting it belonged in the left ear. My heart sank. Her mother, my grandmother, had passed away 37 years before.

An oil painting of mother in a now-faded green dress hung above the sofa upon which she sat. The painting needed cleaning badly. It had decorated all three of the Los Angeles apartments I had lived in with my parents since we arrived from Philadelphia in the early 1950s. "I don't remember that painting, Judy," she said. "Has it always been there?" My heart sank a second time.

"This has been going on for some time now," Mother's physician's associate casually explained when I immediately phoned in to report this exchange. I was so panicked I forgot to ask him what "this" was. And just how did the associate know something about my mother that I didn't? My mind flashed back to a conversation I had with Mother's doctor about her health just weeks earlier. "If I answered, I would be breaking the confidential relationship I've had with Bessie for over twenty-five years," he said. "You'll have to ask her." At the time, I hadn't completely understood or accepted the extent of her memory loss. She was eighty-eight and, like many others her age, an expert at camouflaging an escaping memory.

It was two o'clock on a Sunday afternoon. Mother, who had been a meticulous dresser her entire adult life, hadn't changed since morning, still wearing her blue flannel pajamas and a flowered pink robe. She looked frail and forlorn, lost in the middle of her sofa. I was convinced she was dying. The associate asked if there was any paralysis. There was none I could detect, just confusion and a loss of equilibrium. He asked me to bring her to the office the next day to see her own physician.

I hired a nurse to stay with Mother that night. The next day, I took her to the doctor. But her physician was never in on Mondays; I would have to take her again in two days. I stayed with her that day and although her gait and memory improved, she was lethargic and fatigued and spent much of the day in bed. Looking through phone numbers in the flimsy cardboard box she used as a rolodex, I found the number for Carmen, a caregiver once assigned to Mother when she had refused to call me. Mother had fallen in the alleyway behind her apartment and had taken the bus, bleeding eye and all, to the emergency room a long block away. I picked Carmen up at the bus stop at 6 o'clock that evening and as we negotiated the live-in fee for a week I was, temporarily, no longer as worried about Mother's health as I was about how I would survive the financial implications of her disease.

Mother had always been eccentric. She was born in 1906 in Annapolis, Maryland to Jewish immigrant parents from Russia. Although her first language was Yiddish, over the years she somehow acquired a British accent. Mother was extremely sensitive about her humble beginnings and lack of a high school education and I never asked her about her accent. When friends would ask if Mother was British, I'd tell them she took speech lessons to lose her southern accent.

When I was a teenager, Mother's oversized personality caused me many moments of public embarrassment. Her "Why, dearie, don't I know you?" to a total stranger on the street would send my adolescent shoulders into a frozen slouch and make me want to take refuge in the nearest manhole. Once, on a trip to New York to see the Broadway show *Flower Drum Song*, Mother spotted a Los Angeles neighbor in the orchestra section. Leaning over the third balcony railing, she yelled out the woman's name at the top of her lungs as hundreds of theater-goers looked up in amazement.

So, recent quirks in her behavior had caused me only moderate alarm. On one occasion, convinced that a real estate agent had entered her home at three in the morning to steal her remote control and flashlight, she insisted that the locks on her apartment door be changed. "Judy," she said, "I am *not* imagining this. Do you think I'm crazy?" "Mom, how could you have heard the realtor when you don't sleep with your hearing aid?" But using logic with her eventually became a useless tactic; her synapses were weakening ever so gradually and though I resisted, I needed to understand that the quirks were no longer simply idiosyncrasies.

When we finally met with Mother's physician, he told her that she would need twenty-four-hour supervision and that he would discuss the matter further with me. Privately, he told me to put Mother into a convalescent home. I was shocked that his concern for confidentiality was no longer an issue now that mother was a "goner." I severed Mother's twenty-five year relationship with her physician and took her to a neurologist.

"There's nothing wrong with me!" she screamed in the neurologist's waiting room, "there's nothing wrong with me!" I tried my best to calm her, but nothing worked until she was face to face with the doctor. Mother usually liked doctors; she had the old-fashioned, pre-HMO notion that Doctor is God. Frankly, I couldn't detect any of this particular practitioner's otherworldly qualities. He gave mother a cognitive test: she drew squares, rectangles and triangles and completed simple math problems. She was slow, she hesitated; the strokes of her handwriting, once so bold and distinctive, were weak and irregular but she performed the requisite tasks.

The neurologist asked her a few questions: Who was president? What happened to JFK? What was the O.J. Simpson case about?

"Your mother has Alzheimer's," the doctor concluded. I asked what I should do. "Nothing," he said, "there's nothing you can do except to put her in a convalescent home." I wasn't shocked by the diagnosis, but I was shocked by his lack of respect and compassion. In his eyes, as in the other doctor's, Mother was indeed a goner.

I don't know if she understood the implications of his comments, but as soon as we exited his inner sanctum, she began yelling again. "There's nothing wrong with me, Judy!" "What's wrong with the doctor?" I should have yelled back. And this was only the beginning of our five-year adventure with Alzheimer's.

Faced with the reality of Mother's decline and with the lack of interest of her doctor, I was desperate for information about dementia and for emotional support for both of us. Surprisingly, Mother herself mentioned a geriatric clinic down the street from her home. The clinic had internists, social workers, nurse practitioners, physical therapists and a psychiatrist. It did not perform the miracle I wished for, but it did give me some of the tools I needed to cope with Mother's illness. Visits to the clinic became a valuable source of social interaction for her; the vestiges of her old self were very slow to wither.

Mother called the clinic's internist the "door doctor." "I won't go to that doctor again," she would say. "He's never touched me! All he does is stand in the door!" On subsequent visits, I noticed that the door of the doctor's examining room was always wide open and, although the doctor stood inside the room, he really was closer to the door than to Mother. Jokingly, I mentioned Mother's nickname to the nurse practitioner. On subsequent visits, the "door doctor" began to stand closer to Mother; he even put his arm around her. But despite her pleasure at the physical contact, she still resisted the visits. One day, the clinic phoned to confirm an appointment, but Mother's new caregiver, Angie, didn't reach the phone in time to take the call. I received this message on my answering machine: "Judy, I will not see the door doctor again! Do you understand? I will never go back to him! All he does is stand in the door! This is your mother! Goodbye!"

While Angie cared for Mother during that year, my husband Jaime and I shared that responsibility on weekends. Mother refused to hire a weekend caregiver and when we did, she became so agitated that no worker lasted more than an evening. Sometimes my husband and I alternated weekends; sometimes we would spend the weekend there together. Of course, Mother preferred to have me alone; with her inhibitions increasingly unleashed, she often expressed jealousy of my marriage in cruel terms. Occasionally, my frustration with her stubbornness would make me lose my patience. After one tirade I threw a salt shaker to the floor of her kitchen and we both watched in horror as the broken pieces scattered helter-skelter across the yellow-square linoleum, like the frequent scattering of my mother's thoughts.

The same night I broke the salt shaker Mother was to begin taking Moban, a psychotropic medication to curb her extreme agitation. I was nervous about how she would react to a new pill and uncomfortable about the ethics of medicating her in the first place. To this day, I still wonder what the progression of her illness might have been without any medication.

Months after Angie started working, Mother threatened her with a kitchen knife. I had to leave my classroom to rescue them both. Even with no traffic, the drive between Pasadena and West Los Angeles is forty-five minutes. When I arrived, Mother had already disappeared onto a blue Santa Monica bus. Angie thought she was headed to the Camelot Beauty Salon, but Mother never arrived there. Exactly three hours after my mother's escape, Angie spotted her crossing the street. With psychotropic meds in her system, her gait had slowed considerably. She looked dreadful as Angie walked her to the kitchen: lost, forlorn, weak, similar to the way she looked that Sunday she'd asked if her mother were still alive.

We never found out where she had been but assumed she had ridden the bus for several hours until her thinking cleared and she could find her way home. I phoned the clinic for advice and was told to increase the dose of Moban. Although I continued to have concerns about medicating Mother, my husband insisted we give her the extra half a pill the clinic recommended. Before Mother returned, we hid all the kitchen knives in the baby grand piano. Even with the increased dose, Mother sometimes chased Angie out of the house, but she never threatened her with a knife again.

Almost a year had passed since our life had changed so radically, and by this time we were able to find some humor in Mother's behavior. On New Year's Day, a friend of hers visited and she gave him half of a chicken Angie had roasted the night before. When Angie looked for the chicken to make sandwiches, it was nowhere to be found.

"Bessie, where's the chicken?"

"I gave it to my friend to take home." Mother had been known for her cooking, hospitality, and generosity. She couldn't let her friend leave her house empty-handed. Angie quickly phoned me to share her amusement. I'll never forget her sentence in Spanish.

"*Regaló el pollo*, Judy. *Tu mamá regaló el pollo!*": Mother had given the chicken away as a gift.

But despite some humorous moments, Mother's actions at home had become too dangerous, too irrational and too obsessive to supervise. She put detergent in the sugar bowl, phoned the gas company several times a day when she thought the stove was too hot, panicked about the lights on the control switch for the gravity furnace and disappeared periodically. Several weeks after the chicken made its way into her friend's refrigerator, we moved Mother to an affordable assisted living facility. We knew she needed to leave her apartment but we doubted she would adjust easily to a new environment. On Mother's application for admission into the home, I didn't elaborate about her mounting quirks; I wrote only "memory loss."

She never adjusted to the new environment. When she was in her room, she didn't know where the dining room was; when she was in the dining room, she didn't know where her room was. We knew her stay was going to be short-lived and that another move was waiting in the wings.

Up until Mother's move we'd been able to change the dosage of her medication to fit her circumstances. But now she was in the hands of aides who didn't know her as well as we did, and so we needed to check on her as many times a week as possible. Because of Jaime's more flexible work schedule, he had more time than I did to observe and entertain her. Mother was in heaven during the many drives she would take with Jaime. "You're my boyfriend now," she would tell him. She would even leave him notes pinned to her door, telling him to wait for her if she wasn't there. Oddly enough, she always remembered he was coming to pick her up and each word in the note would always be spelled correctly.

"Bessie's amazing," Jaime would report. "She reads every damn street sign and billboard. She can still read but doesn't know where her room is." Mother was definitely a happy camper in the cozy comfort of Jaime's big, yellow car we called the "Big Banana." If only we could have chauffeured her around forever.

Two and a half months after she moved to the assisted living facility, we received the long anticipated phone call: Mother would have to be moved to a more secure environment. She had wandered seven times in one afternoon, the staff finding her up the street where she was trying to find her brother's home. It had been a little over a year since the Sunday when she asked if my grandmother were still alive. The psychiatrist at the geriatric clinic suggested we check our "baby" into the geriatric psychiatric unit at the hospital associated with the clinic. We heaved a great sigh of relief; Mother would be observed for one or two weeks and her medication would be closely monitored. Then we would have to make the difficult decision about where to place her next.

At the hospital, Mother was calmer and less disoriented. She even seemed happy. I played the piano and she sang. For the first time in her life she wore tennis shoes and warm-up suits the nurses suggested I buy. "My daughter Judy bought me these tennis shoes," she announced to every nurse on the floor. As at the geriatric clinic, Mother soon became a favorite among the personnel. One nurse pleaded with me not to put her in a home but to take her home with me. But finally, at the suggestion of the psychiatrist, what I'll call the Palm Tree Board and Care became her home for the next three and a half years. Looking back, we now know Mother was overmedicated in the smaller facility, but we were not ready to send her off to a convalescent home. Besides, we couldn't afford one. I picked Mother up at the hospital and took her to the Palm Tree. I feared she was going to start asking questions in the car. She was more coherent now that the medications were better monitored.

"Where are we going, Judy?"

"You're moving into a little house, Mom. It was too hard for you in the apartment." I didn't think Mother had any recollection of her retirement home escapades and I didn't know how much she remembered of the apartment where she had lived for over thirty years.

"What did you do with the piano?"

"The piano...?" I stalled. "We had it moved into our townhome."

"Oh, so now you have two pianos." Mother surprised me at every turn. She not only remembered her own piano, but the fact that I had bought one, too.

"I gave mine to Jaime's daughter, Mom. It needed a lot of work. It looks great." We made it to her new home without incident. I just wished I knew what she was thinking, if she knew what was happening. I think we were both very afraid. The manager, Mikal, told me not to linger, so I took Mother to her room and left. I wondered if she had dropped me off like that and then quickly disappeared on my first day of kindergarten. I still picture her sitting on the green, flowered bedspread I had brought for her bed. I still picture her trying to get up to follow me to the door. But Mikal held her, restraining her as gently as she could. While I knew that Mother was protected, as she had been in the hospital, I had given up my control and we had jumped over another hurdle. The lean palm in front of Palm Tree swayed lazily in the early April breeze as we drove away.

Judith has taught French language and literature for 23 years at Polytechnic School in Pasadena California. She has published two collections of poetry, *Shiny Things Make Things Come Back* (2002) and *Lightning Bugs Don't Travel Westward* (2004). Her poems have appeared both in print and online and in the anthology *An Eye for an Eye Makes the Whole World Blind: Poets on 9/11*. Judith also writes in French and Spanish.

Healing Touch

Lois Vidaver

⌒

Daphne loves to dance and often does, right in the middle of the hallway, and it doesn't matter to her whether staff, residents or visiting family members are watching. Petite and wiry, she uninhibitedly trots around as she warbles, "Happy Days are Here Again." She means it. She is a happy camper.

It's easy to picture Daphne before she moved into this facility, the year she turned 75. She still dresses, well, let's say, flashily. Her favorite outfit consists of knee-high red boots, a short red skirt and a white peasant blouse. When she's feeling particularly frisky, she tugs her blouse down over each arm to reveal milky white shoulders. Oh, and she sports a flower in her hair, a big red gladiola. "Come, dance with me," she says, her slim hips swinging and swaying. When Daphne's strength and lively mind were intact, I bet she could have made you laugh and enjoy the party, even if there was no party. But now, if you ask her what she had for breakfast, she'd have no clue. "Breakfast?" she'd say. "I don't know. I don't think so." She is beginning to lose short-term memory.

I have been the public relations director for this assisted living facility for more than seven years. The 120 residents range in age from their late 60's to well into their 90's. Funny and smart, moody and cranky, they are feisty and sweet-tempered grannies and grandpas. To qualify to live here, residents must be able to make their way unassisted from their rooms to the dining room and back and meet their own personal needs. Many still have active outside lives, attending church, going to luncheons and visiting with sons and daughters.

Some, like Daphne, began exhibiting signs of dementia some time ago. Drawn to the front entranceway, looking lost and confused, some wander out onto the patio before they are found missing and corralled. Vera, another resident, is a patio regular. "Is Vera supposed to be out there?" one of the staff members will ask aloud to no one in particular as she passes by the glass front doors. Then she will quickly change direction, step out, and retrieve Vera.

The front doors can be opened from the inside; assisted living residents are considered independent, mobile seniors. One day, Vera tested the system by walking through those doors, down the sidewalk, across a busy street and into a shopping plaza. She wandered, unable to articulate who she was or where she lived, until a store owner phoned the police. She was returned in a police car, where she became "Queen for a Day" to the other residents—they envied her little adventure. The staff members, though, worried. We found ourselves talking at length during lunch about the risks of caring for residents like Vera and Daphne. I often glanced out my office window to see if someone was outside who shouldn't be. Soon after Vera's adventure, the facility's board members and administrators agreed that something had to be done to assure the safety of all our residents.

It took more than a year of preparation and construction before one of the facility's second-floor wings was converted into a unit for 12 seniors diagnosed with beginning to mid-stage Alzheimer's Disease. At its opening, eight of our residents were immediately moved from the first floor into the new wing. I made it up there late that day for my first official visit. As I passed through, the doors to the unit softly clicked closed behind me. Strolling down the wide, brightly lit hallway punctuated with skylights, the first thing I noticed was the quiet. Blissfully, there was no public address system blaring "Miss Jones, extension 308, Miss Jones, extension 308," as there was throughout the rest of the building. Alzheimer's residents do much better in a calm, quiet, family-type atmosphere, a reason the unit is set up for only a dozen men and women at one time.

There was a large printed name card for each resident tacked up on each room door with shadow boxes hanging next to them. The boxes contained carefully chosen mementos from each resident's life: 30-year old family photos, newspaper clippings, and a favorite brooch. I met Lily, who was anxious to show me her new home. "Lily lives here," she announced. Unable to read any longer and using the third person pronoun, she proudly pointed through the Plexiglas of the box at a photo of her and her husband on their wedding day. The photo was black and white and ragged on the edges, but she recognized it as telling her she was home. She invited me in. I looked up at a shelf filled with more keepsakes: framed pictures, an ornate cross, and a pretty vase filled with silk flowers. The shelf in each room is hung high off the floor so wandering neighbors will not walk off with precious family items.

On my way down the hall, I walked past Charlie's room. I saw him lying on his bed through the half-open door. "Taking a nap, Charlie?" I asked. "I should say," he answered, turning his head to glance up at me. "I got up at four this morning and milked 20 cows!"

Family and friends do not often take residents out to eat; their table manners are beginning to deteriorate. Leila's niece is an exception. Once a week she takes her aunt, a former social worker, to lunch. Today was one of those days, but soon after they returned, her niece stuck her head in my office door. "My aunt left this sweater in the restaurant today," she said. "Would you return it to her for me?" With Leila's light pink sweater over my arm, I found her sitting in her chair near the television. "Leila, your niece returned this. She said you left it in the restaurant," I said, handing her the sweater.

"Oh, and what restaurant was that?" she asked. I told her and she thought a moment before answering. "Oh, well, I'm sure it was a lovely affair." It was such a gracious response to cover her inability to remember what had happened a mere hour ago; if she had remembered, she knew it would be a happy memory.

Leila's mood is much like my own. It is such a wonderful feeling knowing our Alzheimer's residents are in a safe environment, cared for by specially trained staff members who will tend to their medications, eating issues and restless nights. The monthly activity calendar posted in the hall lists art lessons, ice cream socials and trips to the waterfront in the facility van. I smile—life is good.

A resident of the Buffalo, NY area, the author has been a non-fiction magazine writer, essayist and award-winning newspaper reporter for more than 25 years. Teaching writing has been a big part of her career, both in the classroom and in other settings on weekends. As communications director in an assisted living facility, she learned to know and love those living with Alzheimer's Disease and feels honored to be able to share part of their story.

Another Dementia

Ronnie Rom

Once when I was in grade school, my father and I made a Mobius Strip together and cut it in two. I have a clear memory of the two of us making a single twist in the long strip of green construction paper and then taping the two ends together. I was mesmerized by my father's enthusiasm and reverence for the elegance and ingenuity of such a simple act: just one swift movement could change the surface of things from an uncomplicated path to a complex journey that never ends. Then, cutting along a line drawn down the middle of the lightly twisted strip would magically turn one loop into an even larger loop that curled naturally into a figure eight, the very symbol of infinity.

Years later, it would be a simple biochemical twist, a mutation of tau protein, that would alter the neurons of my father's brain forever, replicating endlessly into his being and cascading into future generations. "Pick's Disease," they called it. Very rare. "Exotic," the doctor had said. I imagined colorful tribal rites on obscure islands, long dark nights of chanting and head rolling and mysteriously diseased brains. I poured over scientific journals and massive neurology textbooks, dutifully looking up phrases like "presenile dementia" and "inclusion bodies," and "asymmetrical focal cerebral atrophy." I phoned experts and agencies and friends with even the remotest knowledge of such Alzheimer's-like diseases, just to make sure there'd been no mistake.

What was it like to have parts of your gray matter slowly and randomly altered? Tiny neurons swollen and pale like small bundles of useless fish eggs or damaged cherries in a bowl. Were there telltale hissing sounds when it happened, like sparklers hitting water? Could you feel your very self unraveling?

Eventually, the heartbreak of my father's confusion and disorientation became more routine. If asked for an apple, he'd produce an orange; when questioned if he had any sisters, he would mistake the word for *daughters* and answer "two." At a restaurant, he might pour the orange juice into his coffee or, if my mother looked away for a moment, drink the entire contents of the creamery pitcher or enjoy a few choice butterballs from the silver serving tray.

One afternoon I went with my by-then changed father to a confectionary art exhibit at The Museum of American Craft in Manhattan. It was at the exact moment that we were standing in front of a giant chocolate rendering of the *Gettysburg Address* when I realized that my father, previously a nimble-minded Sunday Double Acrostic fan, was pronouncing strings of letters, out loud, as one might expect from an uninitiated foreigner with no recognition of their meaning as words; in essence, he could no longer read.

Since then I've learned that a fair number of Pick's Disease sufferers inherit the disease. Being one who in size, temperament, and appearance takes after my father's family, this isn't good news for me. Like my cousin's wedding table guests discovering that they were not only all therapists, but therapists who were also children of therapists, I find that I now belong to another sub-class of subclasses: not just children of those who have had dementing illnesses, but children of those who have had dementing illnesses who may inherit the disease, or worse, who may pass it along to their children. Or both.

I am a representative of the genetically anxious. We have our own rituals. We sporadically search the internet at odd hours of the day and night, from the National Institutes of Health to the National Organization of Rare Diseases. We seize on vague, disparate, desperate links between *the disease* and lifestyles, *the disease* and obscure substances, *the disease* and nutritional deficiencies, *the disease* and environmental or occupational exposures.

Brains seem far more fragile to us dementia-worriers: complex, delicate, mystifying. I wince when I hear of the journalist who watched a video of his own brain surgery. I crave news about the future of neural regeneration, the architecture of Einstein's unique and cavernous mind, and any insights at all from Oliver Sacks, not to mention the universal applicability of the manipulation of the memory genes of mice! While I fantasize about forming Dementia Worriers Anonymous or Daughters of Dementia, I only hope that my neurosis over all of this will become unnecessary to future generations. Meanwhile, I'm a sucker for any possible connections between the disease and lecithin, aluminum, even dental amalgam. I prod myself—shouldn't I be eating more flax oil or fish for brain food? Shouldn't I be worrying about anti-oxidants, my homocysteine levels, daily exercise?

At other times I wonder: am I having "periodic and noteworthy difficulty with word retrieval" or are my aging neurons simply dying more frequently? Am I "amotivational, confused, disoriented" or does my brain feel like Swiss cheese because I have school age children, a daily commute, and a busy life? Similarly, as my lifelong ideaphoric tendencies seem to intensify, I think, am I like a "dementia victim, deliriously imaginative before her brain begins to show real signs of atrophy or deterioration" or am I simply starved for creative stimulation because I have worked in the same office half my life? At times I want to scream to anyone willing to listen: Is this a sign? Is THIS a sign? IS THIS A SIGN?????

Would my own loving family even notice delicate and subtle differences in my behavior, like so many small pieces of sky gone missing from a thousand-piece jigsaw puzzle, were I to begin a gradual, mental evaporation? But, then, of course, there are whole days, weeks, months that go by when I don't even think about any of this, until a rare moment of distractedly driving repeatedly around the same highway exit ramp loop ... or wandering around in a parking lot. "When you park your car in a parking lot, do you often forget where you put it?" I grilled my husband one day. After his reassuring yet dismissive response, I jacked it up: "Yeah, but I mean every day. *Every day*, or just about? Do you forget where your car is parked in the parking garage? I mean, do you actually wander around the parking garage looking for your car even though you usually park in the same general place? I mean, I've never noticed anyone else actually walking around the parking lot, kind of disoriented, looking for their car..."

During these moments of doubt, I replay the now decade-old memory of my father's face, as we stand together outside in the winter sun, waiting for a bus on the corner of 20th Street and 1st Avenue. By then his fate has long since been sealed. It is very cold, and my father is crying without any sound. I put my arm around him and hold him close.

"I just can't remember! I just can't remember," my father is saying, shaking his head over and over again, as if newly baffled by his predicament.

"Don't you worry, Dad," I say reassuringly. "We'll remember. We'll remember everything...."

Ronnie Rom is a rural healthcare consultant in New England. She has a bachelor's degree from Wesleyan College and a Masters in Public Health from the University of Massachusetts at Amherst. Her writing has appeared in small press publications and national magazines. She is currently at work on a children's novel, a collection of short stories and two non-fiction projects. She lives with her husband, their two daughters and a golden retriever in Western Massachusetts.

Afterword

10 Warning Signs
of Alzheimer's Disease®*
The Alzheimer's Association

Memory loss that disrupts everyday life is not a normal part of aging. The Alzheimer's Association has developed a checklist to help you recognize the difference between normal, age-related memory changes and Alzheimer's Disease. There's no clear line that separates normal changes from warning signs. It's always a good idea to check with a doctor if a person's abilities seem to be declining.

1. Memory loss
Forgetting recently learned information is one of the most common early signs of dementia. A person begins to forget more often and is unable to recall the information later.

What's normal? Forgetting names or appointments occasionally.

---

2. Difficulty performing familiar tasks

People with dementia often find it hard to plan or complete everyday tasks. Individuals may lose track of the steps involved in preparing a meal, placing a telephone call or playing a game.

What's normal? Occasionally forgetting why you came into a room or what you planned to say.

3. Problems with language

People with Alzheimer's Disease often forget simple words or substitute unusual words, making their speech or writing hard to understand. They may be unable to find the toothbrush, for example, and instead ask for "that thing for my mouth."

What's normal? Sometimes having trouble finding the right word.

4. Disorientation to time and place

People with Alzheimer's Disease can become lost in their own neighborhoods, forget where they are and how they got there, and not know how to get back home.

What's normal? Forgetting the day of the week or where you were going.

5. Poor or decreased judgment

Those with Alzheimer's may dress inappropriately, wearing several layers on a warm day or little clothing in the cold. They may show poor judgment about money, like giving away large sums to telemarketers.

What's normal? Making a questionable or debatable decision from time to time.

6. Problems with abstract thinking

Someone with Alzheimer's Disease may have unusual difficulty performing complex mental tasks, like forgetting what numbers are and how they should be used.

What's normal? Finding it challenging to balance a checkbook.

7. Misplacing things

A person with Alzheimer's Disease may put things in unusual places: an iron in the freezer or a wristwatch in the sugar bowl.

What's normal? Misplacing keys or a wallet temporarily.

8. Changes in mood or behavior

Someone with Alzheimer's Disease may show rapid mood swings—from calm to tears to anger—for no apparent reason.

What's normal? Occasionally feeling sad or moody.

9. Changes in personality

The personalities of people with dementia can change dramatically. They may become extremely confused, suspicious, fearful or dependent on a family member.

What's normal? People's personalities do change somewhat with age.

10. Loss of initiative

A person with Alzheimer's Disease may become very passive, sitting in front of the TV for hours, sleeping more than usual or not wanting to do usual activities.

What's normal? Sometimes feeling weary of work or social obligations.

Alzheimer's Disease and a Look to the Future
Maria Torroella Carney, MD

Alzheimer's Disease was first diagnosed in the early 1900's by the German physician Alois Alzheimer. Today, it is estimated that as many as 4.5 million Americans suffer from AD. Patients with the disease experience memory loss and difficulty with thought and language that may continue to deteriorate for as long as ten years, and they can also develop problems with vision, emotions and mood. The course of Alzheimer's Disease is usually gradual; the symptoms may be slow to appear and the extent and intensity of the changes can and do vary tremendously from one individual to another.

Despite the variations however, there are three commonly accepted, general stages of AD that, among other things, are used to help determine treatment for the patient. By testing memory, orientation, judgment, community activities, home life, hobbies and personal care, patients' conditions are categorized as being in a *mild*, *moderate* or *severe* stage of Alzheimer's Disease. In all cases, the course of AD begins with mild memory problems and ends with severe brain damage. Eventually, its victims require almost constant attention, unable to perform the most basic tasks such as eating, dressing and toiletry.

The Stages of Alzheimer's Disease

Mild Alzheimer's Disease

- Loss of recent memory

- Loss of judgment about money

- Has difficulty with new learning and making new memories

- Has trouble finding words

- May stop talking to avoid making mistakes

- Has a shorter attention span and less motivation to stay with an activity

- Easily loses way going to familiar places

- Resists change or new things

- Has trouble organizing and thinking logically

- Asks repetitive questions

- Withdraws, loses interest, is irritable, not as sensitive to others' feelings, uncharacteristically angry when frustrated or tired

- Won't make decisions. For example, when asked what she wants to eat, says "I'll have what she is having."

- Takes longer to do routine chores and becomes upset if rushed or if something unexpected happens

- Forgets to pay, pays too much, or forgets how to pay

- Forgets to eat, eats only one kind of food, or eats constantly

- Loses or misplaces things

- Constantly checks for, searches for or hoards things of no value

Moderate Alzheimer's Disease

- Changes in behavior, concern for appearance, hygiene and sleep become more noticeable

- Mixes up identity of people

- Poor judgment creates safety issues when left alone—may wander and risk exposure, poisoning, falls, self-neglect or exploitation

- Has trouble recognizing familiar people and objects; may take things that belong to others

- Continuously repeats stories, favorite words, statements, or motions, like tearing tissues

- Restless, repetitive movements in the late afternoon or evening, such as pacing, trying doorknobs, fingering draperies

- Cannot organize thoughts or follow logical explanations

- Has trouble following written notes or completing tasks

- Makes up stories to fill in gaps in memory

- May be able to read but cannot formulate the correct response to a written request

- May accuse, threaten, curse, fidget or behave inappropriately, such as kicking, hitting, biting, screaming or grabbing

- May become sloppy or forget manners

- May see, hear, smell, or taste things that are not there

- May accuse a spouse of an affair or family members of stealing

- Naps frequently or awakens at night believing it is time to go to work

- Has more difficulty positioning the body to use the toilet or sit in a chair

- Needs help finding the toilet, using the shower, remembering to drink, and dressing for the weather or occasion

- Exhibits inappropriate sexual behavior, forgets what is private behavior

Severe Alzheimer's Disease

- Doesn't recognize self or close family

- Speaks in gibberish, is mute, or is difficult to understand

- May refuse to eat, chokes, or forgets to swallow

- May repetitively cry out, pat or touch everything

- Loses control of bowel and bladder

- Loses weight and skin becomes thin and tears easily

- May look uncomfortable or cry out when transferred or touched

- Forgets how to walk or is too unsteady or weak to stand alone

- May have seizures, frequent infections, falls

- May groan, scream or mumble loudly

- Sleeps more

- Needs total assistance for all activities of daily living

The patient is not the only one profoundly affected by the disease. The caregivers, who tend to be the patient's spouse but can be other family members, are often subject to physical exhaustion, emotional stress and financial burden caused by the disease. They may be suffering from chronic illnesses themselves and often do not have adult children living nearby for added support. Nationwide, the problems associated with caregiving for Alzheimer's patients are being compounded by changes occurring in the American family, in which both spouses work to support the family, parents have children later in life and have fewer children, all of which will over time shrink the pool of future potential caregivers.

Causes of the Disease

The exact cause of Alzheimer's Disease is not yet fully understood. In the human brain, thinking, emotions, and memories are transmitted chemically along pathways of nerve cells known as *neurons*. At the ends of every neuron, the signal must be transmitted across a space (*synapse*) to the next neuron for messages, such as memories, to be delivered. The brain releases a chemical called *acetycholine* at this *synaptic junction* to help the message travel from one neuron to the next. If a neuron is damaged or injured, or if acetylcholine is absent, then the message has trouble traveling through the brain from neuron to neuron.

Scientists have discovered damaged nerve cells in the brain of the Alzheimer's victim, predominately in the areas responsible for memory. The physical signs of the presence of the disease, first seen by Dr. Alzheimer, are called *amyloid plaques* (Beta-amyloid protein) and *neurofibrillary tangles* (tau protein).

Amyloid plaques are harmful deposits found on the outside of the neurons, and neurofibrillary tangles, composed of filaments of tau protein, are found inside the neurons. While scientists do not know what causes them to appear, the presence of these two substances may lead to a cascade of further injury and inflammation to more and more neurons. In essence, the brain perceives plaques and tangles as foreign bodies and releases immune cells, which serve as the housecleaners of the body, to clear the plaques and tangles away. This continuous attempt by the body to clear the plaques and tangles creates a chronic state of inflammation in the brain that progressively injures nearby nerve cells and contributes to nerve death.

Are these plaques and tangles the cause of Alzheimer's Disease or are they merely the result of neuronal injury and death? Scientists still do not understand exactly how or if these changes kill neurons and how this process plays a role in the development of AD. In fact, there may be many factors that contribute to the development of Alzheimer's Disease. Age is the most important known risk factor: most Alzheimer's cases occur in individuals beginning at age 65 and the incidence increases with age, with nearly half of those aged 85 and older having AD. The number of people with the disease doubles every 5 years in persons over age 65. In addition, brain injury and head trauma may increase the risk for Alzheimer's Disease.

Researchers have found specific genes that confer an inherited risk for AD, such as a *mutation* or gene abnormality, on chromosome 21 of the 23 chromosomes in a human's DNA. This mutation leads to the production of a substance known as *beta amyloid peptide*, a main constituent of the plaques found in autopsies of AD patients' brains. Researchers also believe that abnormalities on chromosomes 1, 14 and 19, known as *Presenilin 2*, *Presenilin 1* and *Apolipoprotein E4* respectively, may predispose an individual to Alzheimer's Disease. Another recently discovered gene, known as SORL1, has been implicated in the development of late onset AD. While it is clear that there is a genetic component to Alzheimer's Disease, this information is not currently being used to diagnose, treat or significantly slow the progression of the disease. More advances in genetic studies are needed to fully understand and make use of this information.

Diagnosing AD

One of the biggest challenges to treating AD is that a diagnosis often comes too late to benefit from the most potentially effective therapies and interventions available. This often occurs because the patient's family or caregiver does not recognize or may minimize the severity of the patient's symptoms. Sometimes the gradual, insidious progress of cognitive loss, along with the development of strategies by the patient to cope with the loss, masks the severity of the symptoms. Then too, family members often believe they are doing a loved one a favor by avoiding, ignoring or making excuses for the symptoms of Alzheimer's Disease. However understandable this may be, by doing this the family does the patient a disservice: the earlier one acknowledges that a problem exists, the more likely a diagnosis can be made and treatment started.

At present there is no test to confirm Alzheimer's Disease. It can only be confirmed upon autopsy. By investigating the patient's health and past medical problems and by assessing the patient's functional abilities, such as memory, calculation, problem-solving, language and attention skills, and sometimes by performing blood, urine and other medical tests, a diagnosis of AD is reached by eliminating other causes for the symptoms, such as thyroid disease, liver, renal or pulmonary disease, vitamin deficiencies, drug or medication reactions, toxin exposures (lead, arsenic and mercury), depression, brain tumors, stroke or small blood vessel disease. The early and accurate diagnosis of dementia is important, because it will lead to appropriate treatment and care plans for the patient and family. Early evaluation of a memory problem has the added benefit of potentially diagnosing other treatable and reversible disorders.

Treatment

The goals of treatment for AD are to reduce disability; to increase independence; to limit suffering; and to manage the disease's behavioral and psychological symptoms such as insomnia, agitation, aggression, wandering, anxiety, psychosis and depression. Treating these symptoms makes the patient more comfortable and makes care giving easier. No current treatment can stop AD. However, there are a number of helpful treatment strategies that have been developed over the last 30 years that can reduce its effects. The oldest involves stopping the loss of acetylcholine in the neural synapses in order to improve nerve cell function.

Several drugs available today, including *donepezil, rivastigmine* and *galantamine* have been shown to slow the progress of AD by protecting acetycholine. A more recently developed strategy involves slowing down the damage to the nerves of the brain. *Memantine*, a drug that has been approved to treat moderate to severe AD, has been shown to retard, but not stop or reverse, cognitive decline in AD patients by slowing down the nerve damage caused by the disease. Although we do not yet know which therapy or combination of therapies might be the most effective, we do have a better understanding of the anatomic and molecular concepts involved which will lead to more effective treatments in the future. With projections of nearly 15 million AD cases in the United States by 2050, it is imperative to our society that we find new and better treatments for Alzheimer's Disease.

Equally important to the treatment of AD patients is providing care for the caregivers. The role of the primary caregiver to an AD patient is extremely stressful. The work is physically and emotionally demanding, unpredictable and lonely and the duration of service is indefinite. To optimize the treatment of AD patients, it is imperative that care givers take care of themselves. This includes promoting their health by finding the time to rest, exercise, eat and sleep well, with the goal of avoiding depression, sleep deprivation and inadequate nutrition while keeping up with their responsibilities. The well-being of care givers also depends on attitude, and learning about the disease helps: know what to expect as the stages of the disease progress; be prepared. As Dr. Larry Wright, of the International Longevity Center has written, "The first rule of care giving is that care of the caregiver is the most effective treatment for the person with Alzheimer's Disease."

Prevention

Many medical professionals believe there are some lifestyle choices that can provide protection to the brain and, in turn, possibly prevent or delay the onset of AD. Regular exercise, good nutrition, including eating fish and fruits high in antioxidants (such as blueberries, prunes and raisins) three times a week may provide improved protection. Participating in social activities that stimulate the mind at least once but up to three times a week, such as dancing, storytelling, doing puzzles or learning a new language may also deter the onset of the disease. Prudent preventive measures to protect the head from injury, applicable for all ages, may prevent the development of AD. This includes wearing a helmet for biking and skating or wearing a seatbelt in a car.

Hypertension (high blood pressure), diabetes, elevated cholesterol, smoking, heart disease and sleep apnea can all contribute to circulatory problems, increasing the risk of vascular injury to the brain. Attention paid to these health issues can potentially reduce the risk of developing Alzheimer's Disease. With the number of dementia cases projected to double over the next 40 years, even modest changes such as these can have substantial benefits for the population.

The Future of Alzheimer's Disease

At present, a diagnosis of AD means a progressive decline in cognitive abilities leading to death. However, there are several radically different therapeutic strategies currently being studied that may bring hope and relief to AD sufferers and their families.

Attacking the Plaques

Alzhemed, a medication in the form of an antibody, directly attacks the amyloid plaques in the brain, slowing the progression of the disease. It is currently in an 18- month Phase III clinical trial involving 1,052 mild to moderate AD patients that is scheduled to be completed in 2007.

A Potential Vaccine

Promising work continues on the development of a vaccine for those predisposed to AD. *IVIg*, or *intravenous immunoglobulin vaccine*, is an antibody product derived from human plasma. It has FDA approval to treat other conditions. It is currently in clinical trials for use with AD patients. The vaccine works by raising the levels of antibodies that latch onto and remove beta-amyloid proteins in the blood to protect the brain against the formation of plaques that cause the loss of cognitive function. Early results show promise for decreasing progression of the disease and even possibly reducing its effects.

Blocking the Production of Plaques

Beta and *Gamma secretase inhibitors* work by targeting enzymes that produce amyloid deposits or plaques. Inhibiting the production of amyloid may decrease the chain reaction of amyloid plaque and neurofibrillary tangle production that lead to neuron death. Research in this promising area of treatment is ongoing.

Blocking the Production of Tangles

Aside from the strategies that deal with the plaques, the other side of the Alzheimer's picture is the tau protein and neurofibrillary tangles. Researchers are focused on designing inhibitors that block enzymes involved in tau protein formation. This area of research has not yet led to drug formation, but the hope is there.

Other medicines, vitamins and herbs are being studied to determine their effectiveness, if any, in slowing the progression of the disease. These studies are looking at anti-inflammatants, cholesterol lowering medicines (*statins*), vitamin E and C (*anti-oxidants*), selenium supplements and Gingko Biloba. None of these substances has been proven effective, but research continues.

Early Detection

Early detection can be improved. One promising avenue is the use of Positron Emission Tomography (PET) scan technology. Annual imaging studies look at the *hippocampus* area of the brain in middle aged and older adults prior to the development of memory impairment to detect changes in mass. Some correlation has been found between shrinkage of the hippocampus and development of Alzheimer's Disease. As researchers learn more about PET scans and are able to clinically correlate scan results with AD, this will become an invaluable diagnostic tool.

More research is needed to learn how to prevent the development, slow the progression and manage the symptoms of Alzheimer's Disease. We need to more clearly understand why and how Alzheimer's Disease occurs and who is at greatest risk. The ability to accurately identify those at risk and diagnose the disease early is imperative so treatments can be initiated as early as possible to reduce the severity of the disease. Society must discover, develop and test new treatments with fewer side effects for behavioral problems in Alzheimer's patients. And it is imperative to provide and find more assistance for caregivers. The time is now.

Dr. Carney is an internist, geriatrician and hospice/palliative care physician practicing in Long Island, New York. She is an attending physician and voluntary staff member at Winthrop University Hospital in Mineola, New York, the Director of the Palliative Care Program at Glengariff Health Care Center in Glen Cove, New York and has graciously volunteered her services as the Medical Editor of *Voices of Alzheimer's*.

Send Us Your Story

Do you have a story to tell? LaChance Publishing and The Healing Project publish four books a year of stories written by people like you. Have you or those you know been touched by life threatening illness or chronic disease? Your story can give comfort, courage and strength to others who are going through what you have already faced.

Your story should be no less than 500 words and no more than 2,000 words. You can write about yourself or someone you know. Your story must inform, inspire, or teach others: tell the story of how you or someone you know faced adversity; what you learned that would be important for others to know; how dealing with the disease strengthened or clarified your relationships or inspired positive changes in your life.

The easiest way to submit your story is to visit The Healing Project website at www.thehealingproject.com or the LaChance Publishing website at www.lachancepublishing.com. There you will find guidelines for submitting your story online, or you may write to us at submissions@lachancepublishing.com. We look forward to reading your story!

Resources

On the following pages you will find information on some of the foremost organizations in the country focused on Alzheimer's Disease research and education and including information on organizations written about by the authors of the stories found in this book.

ADEAR (Alzheimer's Disease Education and Referral Center)
National Institute on Aging
Phone: 1- 800-438-4380
Website: http://www.nia.nih.gov/Alzheimers/Alzheimers
Information/GeneralInfo/

Information, care giving, research information, publications, and resources available; Alzheimer's Disease Process video can be viewed online.

Alzheimer's Association National Office
225 N. Michigan Ave., 17th Floor
Chicago, IL 60601-7633
Phone and 24/7 helpline: 1-800-272-3900
Website: http://www.alz.org

Information on Alzheimer's Disease is geared toward researchers, healthcare professionals, and families.

Alzheimer's Disease Center
NYU Medical Center
530 First Avenue
New York, NY 10016
Phone: (212) 263-7300
Website: http://www.med.nyu.edu/adc/

Programs and services for patients and their families, including diagnostic evaluations, treatment options, psychosocial support and information.

Alzheimer's Foundation of America
322 8th Ave., 6th Floor
New York, NY 10001
Phone: 1-866-232-8484
Website: http://www.alzfdn.org/

Provides care and services to individuals confronting dementia and to their caregivers and families.

Alzheimer's Research Forum
Website: http://www.alzforum.org/dis/abo/default.asp
Inside the Brain tour: http://www.alz.org/brain/overview.asp

Offers a brief description of the disease, including prevalence and prognosis data, areas in the brain affected and the changes that characterize AD; extensive section on disease management; includes an interactive tour of the brain.

Alzheimer's Store
Phone: 1-800-752-3238
Website: http://www.alzstore.com/

Unique products and services for those caring for someone with AD.

Benefits Checkup
Website: http://www.benefitscheckup.org/
Helps people connect to private or government programs that may help them with their needs.

Brigham and Women's Hospital (teaching affiliate of Harvard Medical School)
Michael S. Wolfe, Ph.D., Professor of Neurology and founder of the Laboratory for Experimental Alzheimer Drugs (at Harvard Medical School)
75 Francis Street
Boston, MA 02115
Phone: (617) 732-5500
Website: http://www.brighamandwomens.org/

Hospital noted for its patient care, biomedical research, and its commitment to educate and train physicians, scientists, and other health care professionals.

Joseph and Kathleen Bryan Alzheimer's Disease Research Center Duke University School of Medicine
Durham, NC 27710
Duke Clinical Neuropsychology Service
Deborah Attix, Ph.D, ABPP/ABCN, Director
Phone: (919) 684-3633
Website: http://adrc.mc.duke.edu/

A clinical and basic science center dedicated to the highest level care for patients and families affected by AD and other memory disorders.

eMedicine.com
Website: http://www.emedicinehealth.com/articles/39500-1.asp

Highlights the biological characteristics of Alzheimer's, the general course of the disease and its cost to society.

Family Caregiver Alliance (FCA)
100 Montgomery Street, Suite 1100
San Francisco, CA 94104
Phone: 800-445-8106
Website: http://www.caregiver.org/caregiver/jsp/home.jsp

Public voice for caregivers.

Fisher Center for Alzheimer's Research
Phone: 1-800-ALZINFO
Website: http://www.alzinfo.org/understanding

Five sections (what is Alzheimer's; warning signs and symptoms; getting a diagnosis; where to go for medical help; fact sheets) with answers to typical questions asked by families about the disease and its management.

Focus on Healthy Aging
800 Connecticut Ave
Norwalk, CT 06854
Phone: 1-800-829-9406
Website: http://www.focusonhealthyaging.com/

Mount Sinai School of Medicine's monthly newsletter.

Mayo Clinic
Website: http://www.mayoclinic.com/health/alzheimers/AZ99999
Center locations in Jacksonville, Florida; Rochester, Minnesota; Scottsdale/Phoenix, Arizona

Information on treatments, care giving and taking control; geared toward the general public.

National Library of Medicine
8600 Rockville Pike, Bethesda, MD 20894
Phone: 888-346-3656
Website: http://www.nlm.nih.gov/medlineplus/alzheimersdisease.html

Provides links to numerous government agencies and nonprofit organizations that have prepared overviews of the disease; also links to Reuters and United Press International for recent news on Alzheimer's.

Neuropathology-Dementia

Health Science Research Facility
149 Beaumont Avenue,
Burlington, VT 05405-0075
Phone: (802) 656-2540
Website: http://www.uvm.edu/~jkessler/NP/neudemen.htm

The University of Vermont, College of Medicine two-part teaching module on Alzheimer's; primarily geared for the healthcare professional.

NYC Caregiver
2 Lafayette Street
New York, NY 10007
Website: http://www.nyccaregiver.org/

Local caregiver resource center.

NIH Senior Health-Alzheimer's Disease
Website: http://nihseniorhealth.gov/alzheimersdisease/toc.html

The National Institute of Health web page about AD for computer savvy seniors.

Senior Connections

Francine Siegel, LCSW, Director
Telephone: (516) 292-8920 ext.235
Website: http://www.nassaulibrary.org/seniorconnections/contact.htm

Information, referrals, counseling services and outreach.

Services Now For Adult Persons (SNAP)

Marie Ellen Alberti Galasso, LMSW, Care Giver Program
Coordinator
22702 Hillside Ave., Suite A
Jamaica, NY 11427-2626
Phone: (718) 740-3906

Zucker Hillside Hospital Geriatric Center
Neuwirth Memory Disorder Program

Susan Melchione, LCSW, Program Coordinator
75-59 263rd Street
Glen Oaks, NY 11004
Phone: (718) 470-8100
Website: http://www.nslij.com/body.cfm?id=4961&oTopID=
4961&PLinkID=66

Geriatric programs information.

University of Virginia

Department of Neurology
Memory Disorders Clinic
Paula Damgaard, Coordinator
P.O. Box 800394
Charlottesville, VA 22908
Phone: 800-251-3627
Website: http://www.healthsystem.virginia.edu/internet/
neurology-care/

For the duration of the printing and circulation of this book, for every book that is sold by LaChance Publishing, LaChance will contribute 100% of the net proceeds to The Healing Project, LLC. The Healing Project can be reached at Five Laurel Road, South Salem, NY 10590. The Healing Project is dedicated to promoting the health and well being of individuals suffering from life threatening illnesses and chronic diseases and developing resources to enhance the quality of life of such individuals and assisting the family members and friends who care for them. The Healing Project has applied to the Internal Revenue Service for recognition of federal tax exemption as an organization described in Internal Revenue Code Section 501(c)(3).